Short-Term
Treatment in
Occupational Therapy

The *Occupational Therapy in Mental Health* series:

Short-Term Treatment in Occupational Therapy

Edited by
Diane Gibson, MS, OTR
Kathy Kaplan, MS, OTR

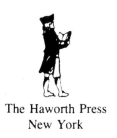

The Haworth Press
New York

Short-Term Treatment in Occupational Therapy has also been published as *Occupational Therapy in Mental Health*, Volume 4, Number 3, Fall 1984.

The Haworth Press, Inc., 28 East 22 Street, New York, NY 10010

Library of Congress Cataloging in Publication Data
Main entry under title:

Short-term treatment in occupational therapy.

    Published also as v. 4, no. 3 of Occupational therapy in mental health.
    Includes bibliographies.
    1. Occupational therapy. 2. Psychotherapy, Brief. I. Gibson, Diane. II. Kaplan, Kathy.
RC487.S56 1984   616.89'1652   84-9115
ISBN 0-86656-342-3

Short-Term Treatment in Occupational Therapy

Occupational Therapy in Mental Health
Volume 4, Number 3

CONTENTS

SUSAN CLEARY SCHWARTZ, OTR, *Program Coordinator, Inpatient Psychiatry, Pacific Medical Center, San Francisco, CA*

DIANE SHAPIRO, MA, OTR, *Division of Therapeutic Activities, The New York Hospital-Cornell Medical Center, Westchester Division, White Plains, NY*

JANE SLAYMAKER, MA, OTR, FAOTA, *Associate Professor, Occupational Therapy Department, University of Florida, Gainesville, FL*

FRANKLIN STEIN, PhD, OTR, *Director, Occupational Therapy Program, University of Wisconsin, Milwaukee, WI*

MARY SAVAGE STOWELL, MS, OTR, *Consultant, Bainbridge Is., WA*

JOYCE WARD, MS, OTR, *Chair, Department of Occupational Therapy, San Jose State University, San Jose, CA*

GERALD WHITMARSH, PhD, *Director of Research, The Sheppard and Enoch Pratt Hospital, Towson, MD*

Short-Term
Treatment in
Occupational Therapy

EDITORIAL

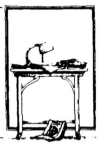

Short-Term Treatment in psychiatric occupational therapy was chosen for this special issue due to this topic's increasing importance and ubiquity. Limited literature addressing short-term treatment is available to our field. Kathy Kaplan, Co-Editor, and I agreed that changes in psychiatric third-party coverage and trends in short-term psychiatric occupational therapy needed review in this journal. I will discuss several prime issues which are based on current literature and my experiences as Director of Activity Therapy in The Sheppard Pratt Hospital.

Alarmed by spiraling health care costs, insurance companies and government agencies have placed payment limits on long-term psychiatric care. Approximately ninety-eight percent of all psychiatric hospital patient days are now limited to sixty days or less. Consumers themselves have doubted the necessity of expensive daily rates and programs which recommend treatment beyond thirty days.

Medicare's initiation of Diagnosis Related Groups (DRGs) in general medicine represents a threat involving further reductions of coverage in psychiatry. The concept of DRGs is that reimbursement for Medicare patients should be based on predetermined costs to treat a particular illness. Hospitals would be paid a set amount rather than actual costs. The threat, of course, is that Medicare and insurance companies following Medicare's lead will pay for less than the cost of present services or present length of stay in intermediate and long-term hospitals. The economic realities upon us behove occupational therapists to validate their services in the most cost-effective manner possible.

Studies comparing short vs. long hospitalization for schizophrenics and nonschizophrenics clearly indicate short-term intensive, psychiatric hospitalization is the treatment of choice for most categories of mental illness. Exceptions to this finding are schizophrenics with relatively good prehospital functioning.

Patient's who seem particularly well suited to short-term care are those whose goals involve restoration to a premorbid functional level rather than those needing reconstruction of basic personality. Patients who are married, who have adequate support systems outside the hospital and whose precipitating event involved a situational crisis such as divorce, loss of job or family member, appear to be the best candidates for hospitalizations lasting under thirty days. Classically, these patients may be admitted when they are suicidal, homicidal or too confused to be able to take care of themselves.

Clinical benefits from short-term hospitalization derive from several commonly accepted program aspects. The structure of the unit environment, as evidenced in a daily schedule, community meetings and activity therapy and occupational therapy groups, assists patients in stabilizing defenses.

The latter modalities focus on reality and discharge planning rather than intrapsychic conflicts. Emphasis of group psychotherapy and activity based groups emphasize increased autonomy, the ability to express feelings, and skill training leading to effective community functioning. For the majority of patients who enter the hospital feeling overwhelmed about their problems, structured activities provide the opportunity to reduce overt pathology and to regain skills. Jackson (83) writes:

> Most treatment is delivered in groups that address common areas of need, such as fundamental task skills, leisure planning, communication skills, independent living skills, and physical exercise. Within these formats, a variety of problem areas may be addressed depending on the needs of the current patient group. Individual services such as, vocational planning, time management, tension reduction, and physical disability treatment, may be initiated as needed.
>
> Discharge planning is an important area of treatment in that changes in lifestyle are frequently necessary. Identifying what changes are necessary and specifically how these may be ac-

complished are within the scope of occupational therapy. The knowledge of available community resources that support and foster work, self-care, leisure, and interpersonal skills should be part of the occupational therapist's knowledge base.

Carefully conceptualized assessment in occupational performance (work, leisure, and self care) and in the performance components (cognition, motor, interpersonal and psychologic) is the key to designing treatment interventions which are compatible with the needs of the short-term patient. Easily and rapidly administered evaluation methods are mandatory. The treatment planning process is conducted on a multi-disciplinary basis and incorporates precise, measurable objectives. Clarity of objectives is important in assisting the occupational therapist in planning and implementing treatment as well as evaluating outcomes within prespecified target dates.

Psychotropic medications coupled with relief from environmental stressors which cause patient breakdown are significant factors in diminishing acute pathology withing the first weeks of hospitalization.

Viewing short-term care as one important part in a continuum of psychiatric care is essential to its efficacy. Brief hospitalization allows staff to evaluate patients' needs, to reduce symptoms, and lastly, to plan for aftercare in relation to patient objectives. Transitional living programs and supervised housing are increasingly important service components which support and ease patients' gradual move back into the community. Without transitional community based programs to support short-term treatment, we can look forward to frequent rehospitalizations.

I hope that the series of articles in this issue will stimulate occupational therapists to broaden their awareness of national health care issues and their impact on our field as well as to clarify the role of occupational therapy in short-term care.

Diane Gibson, MS, OTR

REFERENCE

Jackson, G. Unpublished Description of Short-Term Treatment at Sheppard and Enoch Pratt Hospital, Towson, MD, 1983.

Introduction

The predicted trend toward short-term psychiatric care has become an economic reality. The development of effective psychopharmacology for the treatment of major mental disorders has enabled patients to reorganize quickly. The structured inpatient hospital environment combined with the utilization of multidisciplinary approaches has led to provision of a wide range of bio-psycho-social services for the acute restoration of function. Decreases in insurance funding and increasing costs of health care have resulted in a decline in the average length of stay from two to six months to two to three weeks. This change from more to less hospitalization was initially perceived by many practitioners as a change from better to worse.

However, research and experience indicate that for many psychiatric patients, short-term care may be the treatment of choice. Several studies have indicated benefits from brief hospitalization such as lower levels of pathology and improved role functioning after discharge (Herz, Endicott, and Spitzer, 1977), decreased numbers of readmissions (Decker, 1972), and greater likelihood to continue post-discharge the type of therapy began in the hospital (Mattes, Rosen, and Klein, 1977).

Since the ultimate goal of short-term hospitalization is a successful community adjustment, such as the ability to live independently and maintain satisfying relationships, studies which address predictive factors have particular importance for psychiatric occupational therapists. Many of the studies stress work function and social contact as the factors most likely to affect relapse (Michaux, Katz, Kurland, and Ganseriet, 1969; Strauss and Carpenter, 1977). Symptom reduction is often seen as independent of the level of adaptability (Astrachen, Brauer, and Harrow, 1974; Hogarty and Katz, 1971). Further, the efficacy of phenothiazines notwithstanding, certain psychiatric problems require psychosocial treatment (Keith, 1982).

The significance of identifying predictive variables is clear. Rehospitalization is both stressful and expensive to patients already suffering from mental illness. The ability to focus treatment and resources on factors which most influence successful adjustment would greatly serve the interests of the patient, family, community, and health care delivery system. Obviously, these are complex questions which merit interdisciplinary investigation, practical considerations, and sophisticated research methods.

Short-term psychiatric treatment is one of the most challenging, yet frustrating arenas for the clinician. The demands for accountability, the rapid pace of admissions and discharges, and the range of patient problems require persistent setting of priorities and achievable goals. By the same token, the degree of positive change observed in the patients is often remarkable and quite satisfying. The acute inpatient unit offers multiple opportunities for continuing education, stimulating collaboration, and program innovation.

Occupational therapists are only beginning to realize the potential of their services in the psychiatric short-term setting. In fact, other disciplines have been more prolific in stating the value of the functional assessment (Spitzer, 1980), active and structured group treatment (Yalom, 1983), and the interaction of the individual with the social and cultural environment (Weissman, 1977).

Short-term treatment has serious implications for the role of occupational therapy. This issue marks the first assembly of articles geared solely to the current state of the art. The manuscripts were selected to provide occupational therapists with an examination of the issues germane to their role, common problems, and specific programs in short-term psychiatric treatment. Hopefully, response to these concerns will invite much needed documentation of the efficacy of occupational therapy for this population with clarification of specific techniques, particular outcomes, and theoretical concepts.

Gary Jackson, in *Short-Term Psychiatric Treatment: How Will Occupational Therapy Adapt?*, raises provocative questions regarding the future of occupational therapy with the hospital based brief stay patient. Do the necessarily limited goals of short-term care too severely jeopardize occupational therapy's holistic philosophy and range of therapeutic modalities? Can short-term therapists develop the specialized knowledge base necessary for accountability and professional identity? Will long range planning and greater involvement in community resources establish a role for occupational therapy which is viable over time? These are complex economic, research, and clinical issues which affect the direction of occupational therapy in this area of mental health.

Janet Short speaks to the *Changing Role Expectations of Psychiatric Occupational Therapists.* By examining the stressors related to role ambiguity, role conflict, and role overload, the common frustrations of the short-term therapist are placed in a problem-solving context. The changes required by occupational therapy in the areas of evaluation, documentation, group treatment, meetings, discharge planning and modalities are delineated with suggestions for developing constructive role expectations.

In *Short-Term Assessment: The Need and a Response,* Kathy Kaplan addresses the need for a comprehensive yet efficient discharge evaluation tool. A scheme for organizing and critiquing current psychiatric instruments is provided. She presents an orientation to an instrument, the occupational case analysis interview and rating scale, emphasizing its theoretical framework, scientific properties, and clinical utility. The model of human occupation is used to conceptualize the areas assessed and to articulate the relevance of adaptive behavior for the individual with a mental disorder.

Loring Bradlee identifies the potential of generic occupational therapy groups for assessment and interaction experience in *The Use of Groups in Short-Term Psychiatric Settings.* The flavor of the types of environments therapists typically find themselves is aptly described. The occupational therapists who can adaptively work in this setting are characterized by such capacities as flexibility, realistic expectations, understanding of group dynamics, a system perspective, and a collaborative bent.

Rebecca Gusich's article, *Occupational Therapy for Chronic Pain: A Clinical Application of the Model of Human Occupation,* looks at a specialized program which is becoming more common to short-term inpatient units. The debilitating lifestyles which often result from chronic pain are particularly amenable to description by the theoretical concepts of occupational behavior. A case example is used to characterize an occupational dysfunction and demonstrate the assessment and treatment process.

Two articles, previously published in the *National Association of Private Psychiatry Hospitals Journal,* were included here because of their special relevance to this issue. Boaz Harris addresses each team member's role and the sequence of events from admission to discharge for certain patients in *Short-Term Hospital Treatment of the Acute Schizophrenic Episode.* Alan Levenson underscores the importance of a continuum of services in the mental health care system in which short-term treatment is a part. *Theoretical Issues in*

Short-Term Treatment includes the practical application of crisis theory, milieu therapy, and the medical model.

Marc Hertzman offers a psychiatrist's view of occupational therapy in *A Psychiatrist's Experience with Occupational Therapy in a Short-Term General Hospital Unit.* While the occupational therapy program is designed to assist specific patient problems, several interventions are uniquely described from the unit director's perspective of their impact on interdisciplinary relationships. Similarly, collaborative interactions are examined through co-therapy and in-service experiences. With a balance between specific suggestions and system concerns, conflict resolution, supervision, and professional development are addressed.

This issue has been a little like asking people to bring a dish to a pot-luck supper. Somehow, each person brings something which is different and special, and then the whole becomes even greater than the sum of the parts. Likewise, although there are many contributions, not all the possibilities are exhausted.

The articles as a unit offer a content validity of sorts for the characteristics, themes, and problems common to short-term psychiatric care. Systems perspective, discharge planning, flexibility, accountability, role demands, realistic goals, theoretical models, and collaboration are just a few of the ideas which were repeatedly stressed.

As the authors can attest, the body of knowledge in this area may be experienced by many, but documented by relatively few. The short-term literature would be enhanced by articles addressing such topics as: specialized treatment groups, outcome studies, case studies demonstrating a particular theory or techniques, referral issues, quality assurance studies, and follow-up programs.

Kathy Kaplan, MS, OTR

REFERENCES

Astrachan, B., Brauer, L., and Harrow, M. Symptomatic outcome in schizophrenia. *Archives of General Psychiatry*, 1974, *31*, 155-160.

Decker, J. Crisis intervention and prevention of psychiatric disability: a follow-up study. *American Journal of Psychiatry*, 1972, *129*, 25-29.

Herz, M., Endicott, J., and Spitzer, R. Brief hospitalization: a two year follow-up. *American Journal of Psychiatry*, 1977, *134*, 502-507.

Hogarty, G. and Katz, M. Norms of adjustment and social behavior. *Archives of General Psychiatry*, 1971, 25, 470-480.

Keith, S. Drugs: not the only treatment. *Hospital and Community Psychiatry*, 1982, *33*, 793.

Mattes, J., Rosen, B., and Klein, D. Comparison of the clinical effectiveness of "short" versus "long" stay psychiatric hospitalization. *The Journal of Nervous and Mental Disease,* 1977, *165,* 395-402.

Michaux, W., Katz, M.,.Kurland, A., and Ganseriet, K. *The First Year Out: Mental Patients After Hospitalization.* Baltimore: The Johns Hopkins Press, 1969.

Spitzer, R. *Diagnostic and Statistical Manual of Mental Disorders* (Third Edition). New York: Biometrics Research, 1980.

Strauss, J. and Carpenter, W. Prediction of outcome in schizophrenia. *Archives of General Psychiatry,* 1977, 34, 159-163.

Weissman, M. Assessment of social adjustment. *Archives of General Psychiatry,* 1975, *32,* 351-365.

Yalom, I. *Inpatient Group Psychotherapy.* New York: Basic Books, Inc., 1983.

Short-Term Psychiatric Treatment:
How Will Occupational Therapy Adapt?

Gary A. Jackson, MS, OTR

ABSTRACT. With the increasing prevalence of short-term psychiatric hospitalization, brought about in part by reduced inpatient insurance coverage, decisions must be made concerning both the nature of treatment and who will provide services. The impracticality of traditional rehabilitative services in these settings has serious implications for the future role of occupational therapists in psychiatric health care. It is proposed that necessary modifications to treatment approaches must and can be made without abandoning fundamental theories of practice. Recommendations are made to upgrade the current level of practice via improved communication of information concerning short-term methodologies, to develop long-range plans to strengthen professionalism, and to make greater use of community-based alternatives for the delivery of services no longer practical in short-term treatment settings.

Inpatient psychiatric treatment has been undergoing significant change stimulated by a multitude of forces within and outside of the psychiatric establishment. A new accountability to the consumer and to the sources of funding increasingly demand proof of the efficacy and cost-effectiveness of treatment. The abhorrence of "warehousing" the mentally ill has been mobilized in the spirit of deinstitutionalization, and laws protecting individual rights have narrowed the criteria both for admission as well as for the continuation of involuntary hospitalization. Third-party payers have become a major influence in the provision of psychiatric treatment. To control costs, insurance carriers have reduced the maximum number of hospital days covered and have been increasingly restrictive in determining what services will be reimbursable. Medicare, the largest single

Gary Jackson is an Occupational Therapy Supervisor specializing in short-term treatment for the Activity Therapy Department, The Sheppard and Enoch Pratt Hospital, 6501 North Charles Street, Towson, MD 21204.

11

payer for inpatient services, has recently introduced a prospective pricing system where fixed payments will be made for each diagnosis-related group (DRG). This will undoubtedly have far-reaching implications for the availability of many services. Faced with limitations of time and funding, can hospitals "afford" to provide any rehabilitative services beyond crisis intervention? Choices must be made about what can and cannot be provided that will enable the patient to return to the community without imminent risk of harm to himself or others. Consequently, most rehabilitative services which address the chronic and extensive impact of many psychiatric disorders must take place elsewhere.

Occupational therapists face serious questions concerning the scope and purpose of their services in short-term inpatient treatment. What role is to be played by professionals who have previously been concerned in large part with relatively long-term rehabilitative services? With the rising number of psychiatric beds being established in acute care general hospitals, more occupational therapists are likely to align themselves with the medical model which predominates in these settings. Emphasis on symptom reduction and other short range, problem-oriented interventions may overshadow the more holistic philosophy of occupational therapy. Does this orientation risk what Phillip Shannon described as "derailment" from the essence of occupational therapy (Shannon, 1977)? This appears entirely possible if we modify our approach primarily as an accommodation to the medical model. Shannon further warned that derailment could lead to a loss of legitimacy of the profession and ultimately, absorption of services by other health care professionals. There are few interventions that are the sole domain of a single profession in mental health care. It is not uncommon to find different disciplines providing similar services within the same hospital. It is even more advantageous in short-term treatment to have these multiple options so as to provide a service rapidly and efficiently. It is a mistake to look upon modalities as territory that defines professional identity. This can occur all too easily if at the same time occupational therapists abandon their traditional rehabilitative orientation because it appears impractical in short-term treatment. As a result, occupational therapists would not be members of a legitimate profession. Rather, they would more accurately be considered as health care technicians with an assortment of isolated skills. Occupational therapy services must change in order to be relevant and effective in these settings. Needed change is possible without losing sight of underlying theories of practice. Development or reestablishment of functional independence in major life activities through purposeful activity is a task that unquestionably requires time beyond that of a brief hospital stay. Occupational therapists must therefore begin with direct hands-on service but extend treatment beyond hospitalization with long-range plans that more fully utilize community resources. Occupational therapists are particularly well-suited to assess and select appropriate activities to further treatment goals regardless of whether these are hospital based or whether they originate in the community. This concept marks a shift in the methods used to deliver services but does not alter essential working assumptions. To the contrary, the use of resources in the community may do more to promote normalization of life-style than would be possible by the heavy reliance on hospital-based activity programs prevalent in long-term treatment facilities.

Concurrent with the significant impact that reduced treatment time has upon the practice of occupational therapy, other pressures are rapidly becoming major issues. Accountability will have important implications for practice. Funding with be jeopardized in the near future unless the need for services and the efficacy of these services are demonstrated convincingly to hospital administrators and third-party payers. For too long, occupational therapists have not been held accountable in clarifying treatment principles. Therapists have been allowed to freely explore a wide variety of treatment approaches so long as no harm has resulted. This form of "benign neglect" has resulted in occupational therapy practices nearly as varied as the number of settings but has provided little incentive for practitioners to develop the necessary skills to objectively evaluate their own services. In addition, many therapists practice in "pockets of isolation" (Gillette, 1978). The small psychiatric units in general hospitals often employ a single occupational therapist. This condition precludes the benefit of day-to-day collaboration with professional peers and increases the likelihood that such diversity will occur. The potential for role blurring is great, and touchstones for professional identity must be sought outside of the workplace. At this time, there is not a representative body of literature specific to short-term treatment to guide the therapist. Consequently, the therapist must adapt theory and practice that often originated out of traditional long-term treatment and may or may not be appropriate to this different setting. How to determine what is appropriate and effective treatment has been an elusive issue for occupational therapists as well as for other psychiatric professionals. The problem cannot be resolved by a single practitioner, yet this is the situation that most occupational therapists face when working in isolation. The lack of a specialized knowledge base which is supported by research also does not further the occupational therapists' role as a full-fledged professional among peers and ultimately limits one's effectiveness in treatment. The question is whether or not occupational therapists will develop the skills necessary for effective adaptation, skills central to a true profession.

A blueprint for professionalism was outlined in a special session for the Representative Assembly of the American Occupational Therapy Association in 1978 (AOTA Monograph, 1979). This was not the first, nor will it be the last examination of the prerequisites of a full-fledged profession. Yet, progress towards this goal has been slow. With the demise of "benign neglect," that which will be expected of occupational therapists practicing in mental health pertains directly to professionalism. The development of a specific knowledge base and specialized training in short-term psychosocial treatment, more extensive research, and greater accountability in the clinic cannot continue at a slow pace without serious repercussions. Psychiatric health care is rapidly changing and with it, occupational therapists must upgrade their professional skills or face increased erosion of their relevance within this system. Complacency or efforts to maintain the status quo mark the inevitable decline of an organism or of a philosophy. Is this less true of an art or a science? It is encumbent upon the profession to make these determinations objectively, and in so doing, occupational therapists will also gain the respect and trust of their constituency as well as that of the professional community. The risk is that we recognize our shortcomings, but the potential rewards far outweigh the mediocrity assured by inaction.

An urgent professional need, and perhaps one that may be addressed most readily, concerns reaching the isolated therapist with current state of the art evaluation and treatment methods specific to short-term psychiatric settings. What evaluation methods obtain necessary information rapidly and with a minimum of the redundancy common to multidisciplinary treatment team approaches? Modifications to traditional treatment approaches used in long-term institutions must be made. What is reasonable to accomplish in such a short time frame? Habit formation and the development of major skills are unlikely to occur, but learning effective alternatives to a specific and immediate problem may be possible. Brief in-hospital efforts to improve self-esteem may be insignificant for patients who have experienced years of failure. The value of "doing" is reflected in our philosophy, but time constraints often favor the immediacy of verbal interventions as the expedient approach of choice. To what extent is this consistent with our philosophy? What are the varieties of symptom reduction interventions available from occupational therapists, and in what context are these also consistent with our philosophy? Craft-based task groups may be ineffective in facilitating basic task skills given the time frame, but craft groups may have greater use as initial and ongoing assessments of a patient's readiness to return to major life activities, such as work or school. As previously noted, discharge planning is an extension of treatment into the community where much of the "doing" must take place. The occupational therapist's role in this process should be strong. These are but a few issues pertinent to the increasing number of clinicians providing short-term treatment. A means of compiling and disseminating this information to practicing clinicians must be established. The American Occupational Therapy Association's TOTEMS project to strengthen services in the school system did just that. Their planned development of a similar project in the area of mental health holds great potential for addressing these urgent needs.

A long-range issue for therapists specializing in mental health concerns the profession's role in the changing configuration of health care delivery systems. The unprecedented shift away from institution-based psychiatric treatment and the reductions of inpatient insurance coverage open the door to those who can provide viable service alternatives. Similarly, the limitations of acute care, which preclude a significant portion of traditional occupational therapy services in these facilities, lead to a greater emphasis on referral to community programs. Many researchers believe that community-based models of service, in which facilitation of basic work habits and independent living skills play a central role, may have significant impact on recovery from mental illnesses (Anthony et al., 1978; Beard et al., 1978). The parallels between these programs and the philosophy of occupational therapy are strong and suggest that occupational therapists would be well-suited to work directly within such programs. However, the growth and development of our profession has historically followed its funding. Unless and until outpatient services are reimbursable by third-party payers or other funding mechanisms are developed, this expansion is unlikely to occur to any substantial extent. The strength of our national association and the collective grassroots support embodied in our local organizations must play a key role in securing these funding changes.

Ongoing and comprehensive efforts to upgrade the profession must also be undertaken as a long-range goal. All too commonly, noteworthy accomplishments of individual therapists are developed in relative isolation and remain unnoticed by the professional community. The evolution of occupational therapy services must rest more heavily upon the collective and cumulative efforts of the profession. In this regard, the appearance of the *Mental Health Special Interest Section Newsletter,* and journals, such as *Occupational Therapy in Mental Health* and *The Occupational Therapy Journal of Research,* have expanded the national forum. Not only must evaluation and treatment interventions be given greater exposure, but they must also be validated by research. To do this, graduates of at least the Master's degree level with significant training in research methodology are needed in greater numbers. Even with training in this area, there must be opportunities to carry out research in the field. The premium placed on direct services, particularly in short-term units, discourages the allotment of limited staff time for such endeavors. Increasingly common fee-for-service reimbursement is also a negative factor when the cost of staff time for research cannot be recovered. Larger departments may be more able to "write off" a small portion of staff time for research. Joint ventures between teaching hospitals and universities may be another avenue in this regard. Alternative funding for research, such as grants, must be aggressively sought. The complexities of such a task would suggest that these efforts are best initiated (as some have been) by the national and state professional associations and by the academic community. The subsequent benefits of these activities would strengthen clinical practice and also provide educators with a more unified body of current knowledge from which to teach.

This article has reviewed some of the major changes in mental health care which have significantly reduced the practical application of traditional occupational therapy modalities. Emphasis on symptom reduction, although consistent with short-term care, risks dilution of the profession's essential strength unless brief inpatient treatment is seen as part of a longer continuum of rehabilitation. Active participation in the discharge planning process and greater involvement with community-based resources are effective means for occupational therapists to extend the rehabilitative impact of treatment. Increasing demands for accountability further emphasize the need for research and the upgrading of clinician's skills in the field—formidable tasks requiring support and coordination at the national level. Although many of the newer pressures and limitations in the field of mental health care will continue to be problematic, the evolution of occupational therapy practice may ultimately lead to a stronger, more effective role in a health care continuum that extends beyond traditional hospital treatment.

REFERENCES

American Occupational Therapy Association. *Occupational Therapy: 2001 AD* (Monograph), Rockville, MD: American Occupational Therapy Association, 1979.

Anthony, W. A., Cohen, M. R., Vitalo, R. The Measurement of Rehabilitation Outcome. *Schizophrenia Bulletin,* 1978, *4,* 365-380.

Beard, J. H., Malmaud, T. J. & Rossman, E. Psychiatric Rehabilitation and Rehospitalization Rates: The Findings of Two Research Studies. *Schizophrenia Bulletin,* 1978, *4,* 622.

Friedson, E. *Professional Dominance.* NY: Atherton Press, Inc., 1970.

Gillette, N. Practice, Education, and Research. *Occupational Therapy: 2001 AD* (Monograph), 18-25, Rockville, MD: American Occupational Therapy Association, 1979.

National Insitute of Mental Health. Mental Health Series Reports and Statistical Notes. *Division of Biometry and Epidemiology,* 1981.

Shannon, P. D. The Derailment of Occupational Therapy. *American Journal of Occupational Therapy,* 1977, *31*(4), 229-234.

Spiro, H. R. Reforming the State Hospital in a Unified Care System. *Hospital and Community Psychiatry,* 1982, *33,* 722-728.

Vollmer, H. M. & Mills, D. L. (Eds.) *Professionalization.* Englewood Cliffs, NJ: Prentice Hall, 1966.

Changing Role Expectations of Psychiatric Occupational Therapists

Janet E. Short, MA, OTR

ABSTRACT. Psychiatric occupational therapists have experienced multiple changes in role expectations with the move from long term care to short term care. These expectations have caused frustration, low self-esteem, and job dissatisfaction. These feelings may be better understood in terms of expectation generated stressors as identified by organization theorists. Having reviewed these stressors, this article will review role expectation changes of the occupational therapist in the move from long-term to short-term care and will suggest ideas for adapting to these changes.

INTRODUCTION

Historically occupational therapists had months and even years to treat psychiatric patients. Today, psychiatric occupational therapists are treating patients in a span of twenty days or less. The role and the expectations commensurate with the role of the occupational therapist have changed drastically with the move to short-term care. Feelings of frustration, low self-esteem, job dissatisfaction, and an inability to see tasks through to completion are common among psychiatric occupational therapists in short-term care facilities. These feelings do not have to exist. It is the purpose of this paper to explore the concept of role, role expectations, role expectation generated stressors, and role expectation changes required of the occupational therapist in the move from long-term care to short term care, with suggestions for adapting to the challenge of role changes in short-term care. Short-term care will be defined as a length of stay less than one month.

Janet E. Short was Chief of Rehabilitation Medicine, Psychiatry, in the Henry Phipps Psychiatric Clinic of The Johns Hopkins Hospital when the article was submitted. Mailing address is 1409 Walker Avenue, Baltimore, Maryland 21239.

The role expectation changes noted in this article are those that have been observed in the Department of Rehabilitation Medicine in the Henry Phipps Psychiatric Clinic at The Johns Hopkins Hospital. These changes were brought about by an imposed maximum reimbursable length of stay of twenty days for the medically indigent patient in Maryland.

ROLE

Role is conceptualized as organized or patterned behavior (Lindesmith 1968; Parsons 1964; Sarbin 1954; Turner 1956) which relies upon expectations to define the role and behaviors commensurate with that role (Kahn and Quinn 1970). Role is observable behavior implying action and interaction. Those persons who have expectations regarding the behavior of an individual in a particular role constitute a role set (Kahn et al. 1964). Each day we enact multiple roles with multiple role sets. Social psychologists view not only the interaction between the individual and his role set, but also the interaction of the role and the self (Doby 1966). The individual and the members of the role set are able to judge the performance of the individuals in the role set against those expectations established by the role set.

Expectation Generated Stress

Expectation generated stress is used by Kahn and Quinn (1970) to apply to situations in which inadequacies in the pattern of role expectations prevent the functions of role from being carried out. They have identified three elements of role stress as role ambiguity, role conflict, and role overload (Kahn 1973; Kahn et al. 1964; Kahn and Quinn 1970). Role ambiguity is the discrepancy between the amount of information a person has and the amount he requires to perform his role adequately (Kahn 1973). Role conflict is the simultaneous occurrence of two or more role expectations such that, even if the role occupant has infinite resources at his disposal, compliance with one expectation makes compliance with another more difficult or impossible (Kahn and Quinn 1979). Role conflict occurs not only from externally sent role expectations but also from internal expectations that the person places on himself (Katz and Kahn 1966). Role overload is the willingness to meet the demands and expectations of others, even to acknowledge them as separately legitimate and reasonable, but the inability to meet them simultaneously or within the prescribed time limits (Kahn 1973; Kahn et al. 1964). Individually or in combination, these stressors can create low self-esteem, a high sense of futility, and increase in tension and anxiety, and a reduction in trust of associates (Kahn 1973; Kahn et al. 1964) leading to a disruption in role performance.

CHANGED EXPECTATIONS

Each occupational therapist interacts with multiple role sets daily. These role sets include hospital administration, the occupational therapy department, the unit staff, the patients, and one's own interaction with one's role(s). The expectations generated by each of these role sets can fall into the realms of ambiguity, conflict, and overload which can all affect the occupational therapist's day-to-day functioning.

Short-term care has brought with it its own set of role expectations changing many aspects of the occupational therapists' previous held notions about their roles in the hospital setting. The resulting changes in the therapist's role function on the unit and in the occupational therapy clinic will be explored in conjunction with the expectation generated stressors.

Evaluation

The occupational therapist in the long-term care setting has the time to administer a battery of tests assessing many areas of functioning and establishing long and short-term goals to meet the problems identified. The testing process may take anywhere from a week to a month or longer to collect all the data.

Evaluations in the short-term setting are half an hour to an hour. Information gathered during the evaluation is only that information which can be used to implement treatment immediately. The batteries used in long-term care are impractical in short term care due to the amount of time it takes to give, score, and analyze the data. The therapist in short-term care must know exactly what type of information is needed to place a patient in the treatment programs offered in that facility and be able to gather and analyze it within a short time span. The Occupational Role History, a screening tool developed by Linda Florey and Shirley Michelman (1982) is an example of a tool that can be used and analyzed quickly and with proficiency in its use feedback can be given immediately to the patient. Information gathering time can be shortened by having the patient fill out check lists or other information data sheets while on the unit.

Evaluation is not done only at the time of the initial evaluation. Evaluation is an ongoing process during treatment where the patient's performance is observed and used as feedback to confirm or to modify the treatment plan. Thus, in some situations most of the time spent in a group may be billed more as evaluation than as treatment.

Even though multiple problems are identifiable, time limits those which can be worked upon, and thus the occupational therapist must be able to prioritize the problems to be addressed in treatment. The art of prioritizing must be developed in the evaluation process in short-term care. Prioritizing allows the therapist not only to narrow the problem list so both the patient and the therapist can experience results by working on a few attainable goals but also to establish a baseline of skills needed by the patient before moving on to more complicated skills. Role overload, with the sense that there just is not enough time to work on the patient's multiple problems, is reduced by prioritizing treatment into goals attainable during the limited stay.

Documentation

Initial evaluations, progress notes, and discharge notes remain requirements for long and short-term care. The difference being that turnover is slow in long-term care, thus fewer initial and discharge notes need to be written in a month's time. In short-term care the need for progress notes may be nonexistent depending upon hospital policy, agency requirements, or third party reimbursor requirements. Initial and discharge notes increase due to the fast turnover. More time is then needed for documentation causing role overload as the number of treatment sessions or groups remain the same. There is an increase in the need for documentation which makes it difficult for the occupational therapist to meet both the demand for documentation and for treatment within the prescribed time limits.

With the increase in time needed for documentation, each occupational therapy department should review documentation forms and requirements for documentation. Revised forms such as rating scales that limit the need for writing have been shown to decrease the note writing time and increase patient contact time (Ostrow and Kaufman 1981).

Groups

With long-term care the gradation of groups and the ability of the therapist to move the patient through these groups is enhanced. Eleanor Clarke Slagle (1922) utilized the gradation of groups establishing habit training groups, kindergarten groups, and occupational center, and pre-industrial groups. The patient was able to aquire the necessary skill in each group prior to moving on to the next group. In short-term care groups can be graded, however, the patient is seldom able to move through the various skill building groups due to the short period of time in the hospital.

Because patients are not moving from one group to another, group size becomes a factor. In monitoring the size of groups waiting lists arise. In long-term care patients can wait a few days or a week prior to advancing from one group to the next. The problem with waiting in short-term care is that the patient can be discharged prior to entering the group or that the patient is in the group for only two or three sessions which is hardly time to gain any skills from that group.

Waiting lists cause conflict between the unit team and the occupational therapist. The therapist acknowledges that indeed the patient may need the group but to overtax the group size will only hurt the treatment for everyone in the group instead of just that one patient. Waiting lists also cause internal conflict for the occupational therapist who feels that treatment is being denied to the patient(s). That waiting lists occur is an indicator of the need for more groups, however, the staffing of the clinic may not allow for this. Waiting lists, from an administrative point of view, justify the need for another therapist due to the denial of patient treatment and to lost revenue, an issue that interests hospital administrators.

An issue of concern for short-term care more than long term care, even though it is an irritation to occupational therapists in both settings, is the pulling of patients from occupational therapy groups for testing, interview, and other treatments. The occupational therapist is faced with role conflict with this situation, as the unit team has referred the patient to occupational therapy and therefore expects those services and at the same time expects that the patient will also receive testing, interviews, and other treatments. The simultaneous meeting of these expectations is incompatible and creates frustrations for the occupational therapist and for the patient.

The resolution of this problem needs to begin with the team understanding scheduling problems and the impact of this upon treatment. Agreements can be made as to when patients can and can not be pulled from occupational therapy groups. It has to be acknowledged that the reality of the situation in short-term care is that there just is not enough time to meet all the demands for treatment for the patient during the day. An alternative is evening groups. This is a time that has few interruptions and can be scheduled around visiting hours. Evening work has a great appeal to some therapists who like to work four days a week having a fifth day off.

In summary, groups in short-term care are affected by patients being pulled for other necessary workups, by having to initiate waiting lists to limit the size and to keep the quality of treatment high, and by being unable to utilize graded groups to their fullest in developing the necessary skills the patients need upon return to the community. Quality assurance projects can substantiate that the problems exist and the impact that they have upon patient treatment. Such studies can be shown to department heads and administrators to justify the need for increased staffing.

Meetings

Unit team meetings appear to occur more often and for longer periods of time in short-term care than in long-term care due to the fact that more coordination of the treatment process on a day-to-day basis is needed in short-term care. The role of the occupational therapist has expanded in the team. Even though the occupational therapist reports certain behaviors of the patient in long-term care, the unit staff has a tendency not to act upon them until they noticed the behaviors some days or weeks later on the unit. The unit staff request information and act upon it much more quickly in short-term care, realizing that indeed the behaviors are occurring without their having to witness them. The observational skills of the occupational therapist, along with his/her reporting skills, are expected by the unit team, to give them the much needed feedback on the patient's performance so that immediate changes can be initiated by the unit team.

The increase in these meetings also means that the occupational therapist will be spending more time in meetings and away from patient treatment. In so doing the therapist begins to feel role overload—just not enough time to meet all the demands of patient care. The solution for dealing with the increased meeting time is not an easy one, as cutting out attendance at these meetings means losing valuable treatment information by both the team and the therapist. Sending one therapist to either represent the occupational therapy department or a whole activity department can decrease the amount of time spent by many people in meetings and can increase patient contact time. Another method not especially liked is the taping of important information that needs to be shared. This solution is utilized more within the department than within the unit.

Discharge Planning

Discharge planning and community resource awareness have long been an expectation of the occupational therapist, however, short-term care has increased the importance of this skill and knowledge. The day that the patient is admitted is the day that discharge planning must begin in order that all arrangements are made prior to the patient being discharged and thus maintaining a continuous treatment process from the hospital to the community.

Long-term care responds to many of the patient's problems while he/she is hospitalized, however, in short term care the patient has just begun to work on his/her problems when discharged. The occupational therapist needs a greater knowledge of what is available in the treatment arena in the community in order to better plan for discharge placement. This knowledge takes time to develop and thus places more demands on the therapist's time.

With discharge planning the occupational therapist may find that more time is spent with social workers and other professionals in working with the families of the patients in order to prepare the family to take the patient back into the home. This added expectation can add to role ambiguity unless occupational therapists are clear about their role functioning with the other professionals.

Modalities

Looms, pottery wheels, band saws, lathes, and kilns, modalities and tools that can be found in the clinics of long-term care settings are tools and modalities that should be forgotten in the short-term care settings. Kits are utilized in treatment as there is seldom time to plan and execute a project from beginning to end in short-term care. Kits ordered should be considered for the ability of adapting them to multiple uses and to being able to use different tools on them that will teach new skills. Volunteers in the department can help by pouring ceramic molds and by putting together kits, such as needlework or woodwork, from materials on hand.

Personal conflict occurs for the occupational therapist who has valued the heritage of crafts as a treatment modality but who becomes increasingly frustrated with trying to use them in short-term care. The occupational therapist has the skills and knowledge to carefully analyze and then adapt these modalities to short-term settings and to the needs of the patients.

Other Changes

Other role expectation changes exist. One of these issues includes the role ambiguity brought about by outdated and inadequate job descriptions of the occupational therapist position. Another issue is the feeling of seldom seeing goals fully met as patients are in and out of the hospital so fast. Since patient treatment can not always give the sense of completion and accomplishment, it is important that opportunities are available within the occupational therapy department that meet these needs. Such opportunities include using quality assurance projects that benefit the patient, the department, and the staff, along with staff participating in research, writing for publication, and presenting at conferences and workshops, not to mention presentations within the hospital itself.

SUMMARY

The previous discussion enumerated major changes and role expectation changes. Time has had a major impact on the changing role expectations of the occupational therapist. Time has forced quicker evaluations that are concise and evaluate only those problems that can be worked upon during the short hospitalization. It has increased documentation and may force a different type of documentation to be utilized. Groups are missed by patients due to tests, interviews, and other therapies due to the shortness of time in which to accomplish the team's goals for the patient. Meetings are held more often as treatment must occur rapidly and in a coordinated fashion. Discharge planning, thought of as being done close to the time of discharge, is now begun at the time of admission. Even treatment modalities have been effected by time.

The occupational therapist feels the effects of time most often in the form of role overload. Role conflict occurs due to the constraints that time places on the expectations of the occupational therapist for evaluations, treatment, and documentation. Each occupational therapist must develop assertive skills that can be used to negotiate and define role expectations. The ability to prioritize treatment and use of time is an invaluable skill for the occupational therapist in a short-term care setting.

BIBLIOGRAPHY

Doby, John T. *Introduction to Social Psychology.* New York: Appleton-Century-Crofts, 1966.
Florey, Linda L. and Michelman, Shirley M. "Occupational Role History: A Screening Tool for Psychiatric Occupational Therapy." *American Journal of Occupational Therapy* 35 (1982): 301-308.
Kahn, Robert L. "Conflict, Ambiguity, and Overload: Three Elements In Job Stress." *Occupational Mental Health* (1973): 2-9.
Kahn, Robert L. and Quinn, Robert P. "Role Stress: A Framework for Analysis." In *Mental Health and Work Organizations.* Edited by Alan McLean. Chicago: Rand McNally and Company, 1970.
Kahn, Robert L., Wolfe, D. M., Quinn, R. P., Snoek, J. D., and Rosenthal, R. A. *Organizational Stress: Studies in Role Conflict and Ambiguity.* New York: John Wiley & Sons, 1964.
Katz, Danial and Kahn, Robert L. *The Social Psychology of Organizations.* New York: John Wiley & Sons, 1966.
Lindesmith, Alfred R. and Strauss, Anselm L. *Social Psychology.* New York: Holt, Rinehart, and Winston, 1968.
Ostrow, Patricia C. and Kaufman, Kathryn L. "Improved Productivity In An Acute-Care Psychiatric Occupational Therapy Program: A Quality Assurance Study." In *Productivity Improvement in Physical and Occupational Therapies.* Chicago: American Hospital Association, 1981.
Parsons, Talcott. *Social Structure and Personality.* London: Free Press, 1964.
Sarbin, Theodore R. "Role Theory." In *Handbook of Social Psychology.* Edited by Gardner Lindzey. Reading, Massachusetts: Addison-Wesley Publishing Company, 1954.
Slagle, Eleanor Clarke. "Training Aides for Mental Patients." *Archives of Occupational Therapy* 1 (January 1922): 11-17.
Turner, Ralph. "Role Taking, Role Standpoint, and Reference-Group Behavior." *American Journal of Sociology* 61 (1956): 316-328.

Short-Term Assessment:
The Need and a Response

Kathy Kaplan, MS, OTR

ABSTRACT. Discharge planning usually starts on admission in the short-term setting. However, there are few evaluation strategies specifically designed for this purpose. Current psychiatry evaluations are reviewed, then an interview and rating scale is presented which has content validity and reasonably good inter-rater reliability. The instrument is based on the model of human occupation and expands the case analysis method. Research results are summarized and a case example is used to demonstrate the clinical utility of the procedure. Recommendations based on clinicians' experiences with the instrument are discussed.

Evaluations in psychiatric occupational therapy are at an embryonic stage. In 1979, the American Occupational Therapy Association Annual Conference in Detroit held an institute on mental health evaluations. Three evaluations were presented and supported financially to continue reliability, validity, and normative development. In 1981, the American Occupational Therapy Association Mental Health Specialty Section compiled an index of 80 assessments used by occupational therapists in mental health (Moyer, Note 1). At the same time, 13 evaluations were reviewed and published by Hemphill (1982). The Bay Area Functional Performance

Kathy Kaplan is Visiting Instructor, Department of Occupational Therapy, Towson State University, Towson, Maryland.

This article is based on a thesis submitted in partial fulfillment of the requirements for the Master of Science Degree, Virginia Commonwealth University, Medical College of Virginia, Richmond, Virginia.

Gratitude is extended to the George Washington University Medical Center inpatient psychiatric unit, Washington, D.C., where the study was conducted and the author was employed for eight years. Acknowledgement is expressed to Gary Kielhofner for originating the model upon which this research is based and for his support and guidance throughout the research process.

Copies of the occupational case analysis interview and rating scale can be obtained from the author: 1415 North Hartford Street, Arlington, Virginia 22201.

29

Evaluation (BAFPE) is the only one of these instruments which has substantial supporting reliability, validity, and normative data.

The results of the 1983 Mental Health Special Interest Section Continuing Education Survey revealed the first of the top 12 topics which need to be addressed by continuing education programs is occupational therapy assessment in acute care. While occupational therapists generally recognize the importance of evaluations in clinical practice, they tend to adapt current instruments to meet the needs of their settings. "There are almost as many interest check lists as there are therapists" (Hemphill, 1982, p. 11). This trend reflects a lack of understanding of the importance of using tools which have been shown to be reliable and valid for a designated purpose and population.

One purpose and population for which evaluations are needed is discharge planning for the acute care adult psychiatric patient. The aim of discharge planning is to enable the client to prepare for return to home, or the expected environment, while still in the hospital (Spencer, 1978). During long-term psychiatric admissions, discharge preparation is important because the skills required to function in the hospital environment differ from those required outside of the hospital. While this distinction is also true in the short-term hospitalization, there is usually less of a danger of atrophy of skills (Gray, 1972) due to hospitalization because the length of time away from the original environment is minimal.

The main purpose of discharge planning in an acute care setting is to increase the relevance of the treatment process. Thus, discharge planning usually starts on admission. Optimally, the treatment team considers the inpatient's occupation, life style, and social support system while developing the treatment plan (Dunning, 1972). The goal is to maximize the patient's community adjustment.

While it is critical to begin discharge planning with the initial assessment of the short-term patient, the reasons for admission to the acute care unit frequently render the patient too confused, upset, or resistant to participate fully in an in-depth evaluation requiring paper and pencil response formats. Patients often are psychotic, suicidal, or withdrawing from drugs or alcohol when first admitted. Therefore, the initial occupational therapy assessment may include skilled observation in both structured groups and naturally occurring settings on the unit. As the patient increases in organization and capacity to reflect on the hospital experience, more formal and in-depth evaluation procedures can be used. It is generally recognized that patients are likely to be functioning at a higher level at discharge

(Bloomer and Williams, 1978). In addition, their willingness to explore issues surrounding how they function in the community is usually greater than on admission.

Although discharge planning is a standard part of the ongoing evaluation and treatment process in psychiatric occupational therapy (Smith and Tiffany, 1978), there are few instruments currently available that are designed specifically for this purpose. The Kohlman Evaluation of Living Skills (McGourty, 1979) is designed for discharge planning, but with a population which is generally older or more dysfunctional than the average adult short-term patient. Therefore, there is a need for an evaluation strategy specifically designed for the adult short-term psychiatric patient.

PROBLEM AND PURPOSE

In order to develop an occupational therapy evaluation that has scientific properties and which meets a gap in existing methods, one should consider reliability and validity methods, a theoretical framework for assessment, and the state of current instruments in occupational therapy. Because there is a dearth of reliable and valid instruments for the current practice of psychiatric occupational therapy, there is a critical need for clinically useful evaluation strategies with scientific properties. For the short-term patient, clinically useful means a practical procedure which is comprehensive yet efficient to administer. In this context, clinical utility means an evaluation which engages the patient in self-evaluation and planning and which focuses on components of a successful community adjustment.

The stresses of acute care settings often result in occupational therapists establishing their role by responding to the interests and demands of other staff members. Role blurring and eclecticism often emerge when there is little understanding of or support for the unique perspective of the occupational therapist. Therefore, evaluation strategies grounded in theory provide a conceptual tool for understanding the patient and a focus for the scope of practice.

The purpose of this paper is twofold: to summarize a review of the instruments designed for a psychiatric population and to present the case analysis interview and rating scale, an instrument which was developed to evaluate short-term psychiatric patients in the hospital setting in preparation for discharge. In the first part, a scheme is provided which organizes current psychiatric occupational therapy instruments by type and theoretical orientation. By critiquing the available instruments from the perspective of the needs for the short-term psychiatric setting, a context is provided in which to place the occupational case analysis interview and rating scale. In the second part, the instrument is presented to demonstrate efforts toward systematic development and clinical application. The instrument is based on the model of human occupation (Kielhofner and Burke, 1980) which provides a conceptual framework for examining the effects of psychiatric illness on adaptive function.

OCCUPATIONAL THERAPY INSTRUMENTS

Most occupational therapy instruments belong to one of six categories: performance evaluations, interviews, checklists, rating scales, questionnaires, or projective tests (Slaymaker, Note 2). The current practice of psychiatric occupational therapy reflects five philosophical/theoretical arenas: psychoanalytic, neuropsychological, developmental, functional performance, and occupational behavior (Bloomer and Williams, 1978; Hemphill, 1982). Likewise, occupational therapy evaluation instruments can be seen as representing one of these philosophical/theoretical traditions.

Twenty-one instruments were reviewed which were developed within the last 10-15 years by occupational therapists and designed for adult psychiatric inpatients. Only six instruments were specifically designed for the short-term setting. The summary of each theoretical/philosophical approach is based on a comparison of each instrument in terms of the population for whom it was designed, the type of administration, the yield of the information collected, and the review of reliability and validity data. Table 1 classifies the instruments by type and philosophical/theoretical framework.

Psychoanalytic Tradition

Projective techniques reveal personality features, are generally consistent with a psychoanalytic frame of reference (Hemphill, 1982), and are suited for an initial evaluation of the longer-term psychiatric patient. The type of media used do not appear to have face validity for a short-term adult discharge evaluation which seems to address issues of community adjustment. Although concepts regarding symbolic meaning and defenses are useful in understanding patient histories and interactions, they are not sufficient for current psychiatric occupational therapy practice (Fidler and Fidler,

Table 1

Psychiatric Occupational Therapy Evaluations

	Projective Techniques	Observation: Checklist Rating Scale	Interview	Questionnaire	Performance
Psychoanalytic	Shoemyan Battery a,b,d Goodman Battery a,d BH Battery a Magazine Picture Collage a,b,d				
Neuropsychological					SBC a,d Person Symbol a
Developmental		Mosey Developmental Scales d,e Allen Cognitive Evaluation b,e	*Interview Set b		
Functional Performance	Creative Clay Test a,d *Drawing c	Mosey Checklist *Kohlman d Comprehensive Living Skills b *COTE a,b,d			Activity Laboratory a *Comprehensive Assessment Process a,d BAFPE a,d
Occupational Behavior			*Role History b	Interest Checklist b,d Activity Configuration e/ Occupational Questionnaire	

Note. Instruments may be found in following sources:

a - Hemphill (1982)
b - American Journal of Occupational Therapy
c - Occupational Therapy in Mental Health
d - Moyer, Note 1
e - Hopkins and Smith (1983)

* - Designed for short-term setting.

1978). Especially in the short-term setting, action in the present takes priority over expressing past unconscious conflicts. While the evaluations may be beneficial in aiding the psychiatric diagnosis, an occupational diagnosis involves an assessment of order and disorder in daily living (Rogers, 1982).

Neuropsychological Evaluations

Neuropsychological evaluations for adults utilize task performance to understand central nervous system functioning. The neurologically-based evaluations are often used with chronic psychiatric patients to evaluate functions affected by the central nervous system, particularly, motor, perceptual, and sensory-integrative functions. The long length of stays of chronic patients are factors suited to this type of in-depth, neurologically-based approach. Although some acutely ill inpatients demonstrate neurological deficits, short-term treatment is generally incompatible with neurologic reintegrative approaches.

Developmental Evaluations

Evaluations from a developmental frame of reference for the adult psychiatric patient stress the sequential acquisition of adaptive skills required for effective interaction with the environment. A wide range of physical and psychological abilities are considered interdependent and necessary for adaptive functioning. In the short-term setting, the appreciation of developmental factors is critical in correctly understanding an individual's current situations. However, decisions need to be made about which abilities are most crucial to evaluate for a given individual because of time factors.

Functional Performance

A fourth group of psychiatric evaluations relate to functional behavior in work, leisure, or self-care activities. The typical conceptual model behind these assessments proposes that skills are acquired through practice and reinforcement (Mosey, 1970, 1973). Observation checklists and rating scales provide objective means for measuring behavior. These are commonly used to assess functioning in activities of daily living and are relevant to the needs of patients close to discharge. The performance evaluation also provides a wealth of information about functional skills. Sometimes, additional information is needed to prepare a patient adequately for discharge, such as the way in which skills are supported by the individual's expected environment.

Occupational Behavior Evaluations

The final category of psychiatric evaluations reflects those based on occupational behavior theory. Occupational behavior is based on the early concepts of the field, such as the importance of a balance among work, play, rest, and sleep (Meyer, 1922); the development of skills necessary for productive role performance which are integrated into habitual routines (Heard, 1977; Slagle, 1922); and the notion that adaptation requires the satisfaction of both internal and external expectations for performance and interaction with the environment for the person to be effective and experience a sense of personal control (Burke, 1977; Moorehead, 1969).

The relevance of occupational behavior theory to psychiatric occupational therapy is exemplified by the psychiatric literature on adaptation and community adjustment in which the conceptualization of what is necessary for normal function and mental health is based on examining the individual in interaction with his social and cultural environment (Hogarty and Katz, 1971; Weissman, 1975). In addition, the increasing recognition of the limitations of psychopharmocology in treating some functional abilities and characteristic problems such as "the lack of goal directed behavior, profound associability, [and] the absence of affectual drive" (Keith, 1982, p. 793), points to the importance of psychosocial treatment approaches which address adaptive functional behavior.

An occupational therapy research project by Fran Oakley (Note 2), at the National Institute of Mental Health, Washington, D.C., specifically addresses the relevance of the model of human occupation to psychiatry. She evaluated 30 male and female adult hospitalized patients (mostly diagnosed as depressed or schizophrenic) with eight instruments to determine the relationship of the organizational status of the human system to adaptive level of functioning, degree of symptomatology, past psychiatric history, and past productivity. Organizational status was derived from a clinician's blind rating of all the evaluation data, translating it into a single score on a five point continuum from very organized to very disorganized. Oakley's data analysis revealed a high correlation between the organizational status of the human system and adaptive level of functioning. Organizational status was inversely related to past psychiatric history and degree of symptomatology; however, the correlation was not high enough to argue that organizational status was primarily a function of symptomatology. Rather, data revealed that organizational status was a better indicator of adaptive functioning than diagnoses or symptomatology.

Research such as the above allows occupational therapists to identify and substantiate their contribution to psychiatric care more clearly. This is why the model of occupation is the framework from which this discharge evaluation is derived. The occupational behavior evaluations are conceptually similar to the theory base of the proposed discharge evaluation, but they do not provide an organized way to gather information from each component of the model of human occupation as it applies to short-term patients. Therefore, the development of the occupational case analysis interview and rating scale is an effort to begin the process of instrumentation which fills a gap in the evaluations available for the short-term psychiatric adult inpatient.

THE OCCUPATIONAL CASE ANALYSIS INTERVIEW AND RATING SCALE

The case analysis method (Cubie and Kaplan, 1982) was developed as a way to bridge theory from the model of human occupation (Kielhofner and Burke, 1980) to clinical practice. That method is comprised of ten primary questions derived from the model of human occupation and four questions regarding the global assessment of the overall system which provide a method for analyzing clinical cases and assessing an individual's overall trajectory. The case analysis interview was developed to yield information for each of 14 identified model concepts and to serve as a screening discharge evaluation for acute care psychiatric adult patients. The case analysis rating scale provides an objective method of measuring adaptive behavior by assigning a five point ordinal rating for each primary question and system analysis. For each concept, ratings are between 1 and 5, with 5 representing the most adaptive behavior and 1 representing the least adaptive behavior. A portion of the instrument is presented in Table 2. There is also a separate summary form for recording scores and comments for each patient interviewed which is seen in the case example section.

Table 2

Occupational Case Analysis Interview and Rating Scale
Post-Research Version

MODEL COMPONENTS AND PRIMARY QUESTIONS	INTERVIEW QUESTIONS:	RATING SCALE AND GUIDELINES
INTERESTS: Does the individual have interests?	a. How do you like to spend your time?	III. INTERESTS (leisure, Work Related (etc.)) 5. Identifies a variety (four or more) of satisfying interests; two activities pursued regularly
YIELD: to identify interests and frequency of participation	b. Do you have any other special interests?	4. Identifies a variety of satisfying interests; participation is variable 3. Identifies a few (one to three) interests; one activity pursued regularly
	c. How often do you participate?	2. Identifies a few interests; participation is variable 1. Does not identify any interests.
ROLES: Does the individual have a primary occupational role?	a. How do you describe yourself, when people ask you what to do?	IV. ROLES (Worker, Caretaker, etc.) 5. Realistically describes many (five or more) activities or obligations of a primary role.
YIELD: to identify activities of one role, in detail	b. What kind of responsibilities do you have as a ___? (fill in from previous response)	4. Realistically describes several (three-four) activities or obligations of a primary role. 3. Realistically describes one or two activities or obligations of a primary role.
		2. Somewhat realistically (or vaguely) describes the activities or obligations of a primary role. 1. Does not describe a primary role.

Methods and Results

The instrument was developed in two phases. To determine content validity, the instrument was submitted to a panel of experts, and to determine inter-rater reliability, four trained occupational therapists rated nine videotaped interviews of adult psychiatric inpatients. The patients were hospitalized on the 34-bed inpatient unit of George Washington University Medical Center. The average length of stay is two to three weeks. The patients, identified through chart review and psychiatrist recommendation, met the following criteria: (1) patients between ages 19 and 60; (2) carrying a diagnosis of depression or schizophrenia (excluding schizoaffective disorders); (3) hospitalized at least 4 days or demonstrating organized behavior; and (4) giving written consent to be videotaped for participation in the study after full information was provided.

The feedback from the experts suggested that the content of the instrument was valid. Inter-rater reliability, as assessed using intraclass correlation coefficient (ICC), was reasonably good for the majority of individual component ratings and strongest for the instrument total score (Table 3).

ICC is an appropriate measure for estimating the reliability of quantitative data (Bartko, 1966; Bartko and Carpenter, 1976; Fleiss, 1975; Fleiss and Cohen, 1973). Correlation coefficients express the degree of relationship between two variables. In order to compute the ICC, an analysis of variance is done to estimate the components of variability in the statistic model for the data, i.e., subject and error. Landis and Koch (1977) state that, under certain realistic conditions, the weighted Kappa statistic is essentially equivalent to the ICC. Since there are no published guidelines for the meaning of the ICC, information about weighted Kappa was used as a guideline. Landis and Koch (1977) offer the following labels when describing the strength of agreement which corresponds with these ranges of Kappa statistics:

Kappa Statistic	Strength of Agreement
≤ 0.00	Poor
0.00 - 0.20	Slight
0.21 - 0.40	Fair
0.41 - 0.60	Moderate
0.61 - 0.80	Substantial
0.81 - 1.00	Almost Perfect

Table 3

Intraclass Correlation Coefficients

Components:	Almost Perfect	Substantial	Moderate	Fair
Personal Causation			.511	
Values/Goals		.672		
Interests	.812			
Internalized Roles	.948			
Habit Patterns		.766		
Skills		.728		
Output		.758		
Physical Environment			.594	
Social Environment	.828			
Feedback				.403
Global Assessment:				
Dynamic		.691		
Historical			.567	
Contextual		.630		
System Trajectory				.318
Component Total	.882			
Global Assessment Total		.744		
Instrument Total	.893			
	0.81-1.00	0.61-0.80	0.41-0.60	0.21-0.40

In addition, analysis of the relationship between the sum of component ratings and the sum of global assessment ratings was done. The Pearson product-moment correlation coefficients ranged from .801-.951, and were all significant at the .01 level. Based on the statistical results and descriptive data from the raters, the instrument was revised into the post-research version.

CASE EXAMPLE

M. is a 35 year old male who was admitted to the unit due to suicidal thoughts. He had been separated from his wife, working long hours, and experiencing weight loss and lack of sleep. Currently, he was staying with a friend while his wife lived with their daughter at their home. He had worked his way up an organization over 17 years and was presently a salesman. He had a bachelor of science degree in business with vague plans to get a masters degree in finance.

During the 20 minute interview, the patient answered questions readily, although mood and affect were depressed. The interview revealed a person with role imbalance who had difficulty forming goals which would enable him to make changes. He desired more leisure time and more satisfaction with interpersonal relationships. While problem-solving skills regarding work were excellent, they were not adequately applied to other parts of his life. Family and friends were available for support, but lacked understanding about his emotional turmoil.

Discharge planning involved getting additional information about values and interests, helping patient set goals and make specific plans, and identifying a support system which could help the patient apply more effective coping skills to interpersonal relationships to ultimately develop more satisfaction with his life. The assessment is summarized in Table 4.

Meaning of Ratings

Most of this patient's scores were rated a 3, indicating moderately maladaptive functioning. Had only skills been evaluated, he would look like a high functioning patient. The advantage of the occupational case analysis interview is that other areas are given priority, such as, how skills are organized into routines which support role behavior; the effect of the environment on expectations and performance; and the interplay of one's anticipation of success, identification of interests, and specification of goals.

When, as in the global assessments, the interaction of the components are considered together and compared with how the patient has functioned over time, the overall impression, or system trajectory, can be more dysfunctional. This patient's total score was the fourth highest out of the nine patients interviewed in the original

Table 4

Occupational Case Analysis Interview and Rating Scale: Summary Form

Patient: M.		Rater: KK	Date: 7/12/83
DATA ANALYSIS			
Model Components	Rating 5-1	Summary Comments	
I. Personal Causation	3	Feels successful about work but unsuccessful about personal life	
II. Valued Goals	3	Values staying alive, but has no specific goals, vague plans	
III. Interests	3	Identifies 3 interests (golf, bike, hikes) golfs once a week	
IV. Internalized Roles	4	Realistically describes 3-4 activities of work role - sales manager	
V. Habit Patterns	4	Pretty well organized daily schedule, but no leisure activities	
VI. Skills	4	Excellent work skills, needs improvement in leisure and personal relationships	
VII. Output	3	Not very satisfied, works but no leisure	
VIII. Physical Environment	5	No problems mentioned	
IX. Social Environment	3	Give advice, he should be happy with what he has, they do not understand his turmoil	
X. Feedback	3	Self-reflection, attempts to change but not successful	
SYSTEM ANALYSIS - Global Assessments			
XI. Dynamic	3	Habits and role in contradiction to volition; identifies desire to change	
XII. Historical	3	In pain now, but marital separation was worse, some good times in past	
XIII. Contextual	3	(Unrealized) goals and performance somewhat congruent with environmental expectations	
XIV. System Trajectory	2	Recurring maladaptive cycle, needs help to reorganize	
XV. TOTAL: (14-70 range)	46	RECOMMENDATIONS: Needs help to be specific about identifying plans, goals, and values. Needs to expand interests and practice to integrate leisure into daily routine. Develop interpersonal and self-assessment skills. Strengths in process, motor, and work skills and ability to organize and desire to change. Long term goals: balance between work and leisure and relationships; increased personal causation.	

sample. Yet, his ratings on personal causation and valued goals were some of the lowest.

In general, a patient who is very resistant to being interviewed may receive mostly ratings of 1, indicating a true assessment cannot be determined. Some patients may have a very mixed picture, for example, with 5 ratings in personal causation and interest, but 2 ratings in feedback and historical assessments. Not only is the rating for each component variable for each individual, but also the way a component affects an individual's sense of self, lifestyle satisfaction, actual occupational behavior, and significant others is unique. It is the comprehensiveness and sensitivity of this screening assessment, based on occupational behavior theory and applied to individual clinical cases, that is its major strength.

DISCUSSION

Clinicians who were involved in the development of the instrument have used the instrument and have found it beneficial with certain patients. Patients who were considering major changes and hence in need of careful discharge planning and were also able to articulate their concerns sufficiently in an interview, were seen as most appropriate for this assessment process. Therapists reported that the sequence of questions seemed to quickly establish rapport, and patients found the process itself instructive. The comprehensive nature helped to paint a picture of a patient's strengths and weaknesses, and the treatment plan followed logically. Areas which needed further evaluation were easily identified.

An additional benefit was the way in which the content of the instrument facilitated team functioning. The occupational therapists were more sensitive to information gathered by other team members such as data regarding family members and the environment. Likewise, the role of the occupational therapist was strengthened by using this framework for eliciting and reporting clinical information.

Once therapists were comfortable with the instrument, they could make the ratings and record the summary information in about 20 minutes. Documenting the ratings and comments on the summary form provided an efficient way to present a great deal of information which was easy to read and which served to objectify clinical judgment.

Suggestions for improving the instrument included writing a manual to assist with decision-making and applying theory to treatment/discharge planning. In order to use the instrument reliably, the therapist must have background familiarity with the model of human occupation and the case analysis method. A limitation of the assessment is that it relies on self-report and interviewer skill. Therefore, additional information from observation in groups or other evaluations may improve the validity of the results.

SUMMARY AND RECOMMENDATIONS

The statistical results of this study suggest that the occupational case analysis interview and rating scale has fairly good inter-rater reliability and content validity. While correlation coefficients for some items were less than desirable, inter-rater reliability suggests that a trained therapist can use the interview and rating scale to objectively measure each of the components of the occupational case analysis method as it relates to the adult psychiatric patient.

The current instrument would benefit from other studies of reliability and the collection of normative data. Additional studies are necessary to establish the usefulness of the instrument in measuring adaptive functioning and predicting successful community adjustment. In order to determine the meaning of the scores based on theory from the model of human occupation, studies of construct validity are needed. Continued suggestions for revision are necessary from short-term therapists who use the instrument and can address its clinical utility.

Short-term psychiatric occupational therapists need reliable and valid instruments specially designed for acute settings. The occupational case analysis interview and rating scale appears to provide a consistent measure with content validity for a discharge planning instrument based on the model of human occupation. The instrument gathers and organizes a great deal of information in a relatively short amount of time, and it reflects the beginning stage of instrument development for evaluation of the factors necessary for successful community adjustment.

REFERENCE NOTES

1. Moyer, E. *Index of Assessments Used by Occupational Therapists in Mental Health.* American Occupational Therapy Association Special Interest Group, 1981.

2. Oakley, F. *The Model of Human Occupation in Psychiatry.* Unpublished Masters Research Project, Virginia Commonwealth University, 1982.

3. Slaymaker, J. *Results of Mental Health Task Force*. Presentation at the Mental Health Assessment Institute, American Occupational Therapy Association Annual Conference, Detroit, April 21, 1979.

BIBLIOGRAPHY

Bartko, J. The intraclass correlation coefficient as a measure of reliability. *Psychological Reports*, 1966, *19*, 3-11.

Bartko, J. and Carpenter, W. On the methods and theory of reliability. *The Journal of Nervous and Mental Disease*, 1976, 163, 307-317.

Bloomer, J. and Williams, S. *Bay Area Functional Performance Evaluation* (Research ed.). Palo Alto, California: Consulting Psychologists Press, 1978.

Burke, J. A clinical perspective on motivation: Pawn versus origin. *American Journal of Occupational Therapy*, 1977, 31, 254-259.

Cubie, S. and Kaplan, K. A case analysis method for the model of occupation. *American Journal of Occupational Therapy*, 1982, *36*, 645-656.

Dunning, H. Environmental occupational therapy. *American Journal of Occupational Therapy*, 1972, *26*, 92-298.

Fidler, G. and Fidler, J. Doing and becoming: Purposeful action and self-actualization. *American Journal of Occupational Therapy*, 1978, *32*, 305-310.

Fleiss, J. Measuring agreement between two judges on the presence or absence of a trait. *Biometrics*, 1975, *31*, 651-659.

Fleiss, J. and Cohen, J. The equivalence of weighted Kappa and the intraclass correlation coefficient as measures of reliability. *Educational and Psychological Measurement*, 1973, *33*, 613-619.

Gray, M. The effects of hospitalization on work-play behavior. *American Journal of Occupational Therapy*, 1972, *26*, 180-185.

Heard, C. Occupational role acquisition: A perspective on the chronically disabled. *American Journal of Occupational Therapy*, 1977, *31*, 243-247.

Hemphill, B. *Evaluation Process in Psychiatric Occupational Therapy*. New Jersey: Charles B. Slack, 1982(b).

Hogarty, G. and Katz, M. Norms of adjustment and social behavior. *Archives of General Psychiatry*, 1971, 25, 470-480.

Keith, S. Drugs: not the only treatment. *Hospital and Community Psychiatry*, 1982, *33*, 793.

Kielhofner, G. and Burke, J. A model of human occupation, part 1, conceptual framework and content. *American Journal of Occupational Therapy*, 1980, *34*, 572-581. (d)

Kielhofner, G. and Burke, J. Occupational therapy after 60 years: An account of changing identity and knowledge. *American Journal of Occupational Therapy*, 1977, *31*, 675-688.

Landis, J. and Koch, G. The measurement of observer agreement for categorical data. *Biometrics*, 1977, *33*, 159-174.

McGourty, L. *Kohlman Evaluation of Living Skills*. Seattle, Washington: KELS Research, 1979.

Meyer, A. The philosophy of occupational therapy. *Archives of Occupational Therapy*, 1922, *1*, 1-10.

Moorehead, L. The occupational history. *American Journal of Occupational Therapy*, 1969, *23*, 329-334.

Mosey, A. *Activity Therapy*. New York: Raven Press, 1973.

Mosey, A. *Three Frames of Reference for Mental Health*. New Jersey: Charles B. Slack, 1970.

Rogers, J. Order and disorder in medicine and occupational therapy. *American Journal of Occupational Therapy*, 1982, *36*, 29-35.

Slagle, E. Training aids for mental patients. *Occupational Therapy and Rehabilitation*, 1922, *1*, 11-17.

Smith, H. and Tiffany, E. Assessment and evaluation. In H. Hopkins and H. Smith (eds.), *Willard and Spackman's Occupational Therapy* (Fifth Edition). Philadelphia: J.B. Lippincott Company, 1978.

Spencer, E. Functional restoration. In H. Hopkins and H. Smith (eds.), *Willard and Spackman's Occupational Therapy* (Fifth Edition). Philadelphia: J.B. Lippincott Company, 1978.

Weissman, M. Assessment of social adjustment. *Archives of General Psychiatry,* 1975, *32,* 351-365.

The Use of Groups in Short-Term Psychiatric Settings

Loring Bradlee, MS, OTR

ABSTRACT. This paper will examine the use of occupational therapy groups in short-term psychiatric settings. Included will be an overview of the use of groups in psychiatry, a consideration of the characteristic features of a short-term unit, a discussion of the purposes of the occupational therapy group and an explanation of the interplay between the occupational therapy group and the therapeutic milieu. In addition, there will be a description of points to be considered in developing an occupational therapy group on a short-term unit.

The last two decades have witnessed significant changes in the nature and provision of occupational therapy services in psychiatric settings. Some of these changes reflect internal developments within the profession of occupational therapy while others reflect changing trends in the field of psychiatry at large. With specific regard to inpatient treatment, certainly the trend has been toward time-limited hospitalization. As stated by Crory, Sebastian and Mosey (1974), "short-term, in-hospital patient treatment is a reality brought on in part by rising hospitalization costs, more effective somatic treatment, and movement toward community-based treatment" (p. 401). This trend is based upon both clinical and fiscal considerations. In some instances, psychiatric hospitals once associated with longer-term care have dramatically shortened their average length of stay. In other instances, general hospitals have opened their own short-term psychiatric units. It has been noted that while in the

Loring Bradlee is a graduate of the Basic Professional Master's Program at B.U.'s Sargent College. She has worked in short-term inpatient psychiatry for eight years, most recently at the VA Hospital in White River Junction, Vermont. She is currently pursuing an M.B.A. in Health Care Management at Boston University.

1940's there were only a few dozen such units, there are now as many as 1,700 (Sederer, 1983).

In the context of these changes, occupational therapists have been faced with the challenge of developing treatment programs that are both appropriate to short-term inpatient settings and effective in facilitating adaptive functioning. The decision to adopt a group format is often based on the therapist's own treatment philosophy, the purposes of the program, and logistical factors such as staffing patterns. Historically, occupational therapists have tended to rely upon a group orientation in the psychiatric services they provided. Consider, however, the contrast between developing a group program for a contemporary short-term unit where the average stay is a matter of weeks with a program described in a 1955 AJOT article entitled "Activity Group Therapy" in which the group membership extended for two years (Bobis, Harrison, & Traub). Additionally, there appears to be a shift away from the almost exclusively schizophrenic population reflected in this early literature to a more varied diagnostic population which often contains individuals of a higher functional level.

In developing group-oriented programs to coincide with these trends, occupational therapists have undoubtedly responded in a myriad of ways dependent in part on their own training and academic background. Some retain a traditional reliance on craft activities while others have expanded into areas of self-expression and communication skills. Some emphasize stress management while others concentrate on daily living skills. Some may stress physical modalities while others rely on cognitive strategies. Given such variation, how can one meaningfully consider such groups in terms of a larger spectrum?

To establish this broader perspective, it seems that several considerations may be necessary. First, there is the need to examine our own professional heritage in regard to the use of groups in psychiatric treatment. Secondly, there is the need to explore the specific features that are unique to the nature of inpatient units and that therefore impact on treatment programs operating within. Thirdly, there is the consequent need to look at the kinds of considerations and adaptations that may be indicated in developing group programs for short-term psychiatric settings.

The literature contains some record of efforts to conceptualize the use of groups in psychiatric occupational therapy. Shannon and Snortun (1965) proposed that "by working in a group of limited size, the patient could be provided with a more closely supervised opportunity for practicing rudimentary social skills and receive needed feedback from actual experience, thereby discovering that he is capable of handling social situations that formerly prompted his withdrawal'' (p. 345). These fundamentals are expanded and elaborated by Gail Fidler in her hallmark 1969 article ''The Task-Oriented Group As a Context for Treatment.'' In this she postulates that

> the intent of the task-oriented group is to provide a shared working experience wherein the relationship between feeling, thinking and behavior, their impact on others and task accomplishment can be viewed and explored. Task accomplishment is seen as the catalytic agent which elicits behavior and interaction, brings into focus both functional capacities and limitations, facilitates collaboration in working through problems and provides a concrete reality against which to measure learning and achievement (p. 45).

Subsequently, in her article ''The Concept and Use of Developmental Groups,'' published in the following year, Anne Mosey outlined her developmental theory of groups which suggests that group-oriented programs should be graded so as to facilitate the acquisition of interactional skills. These skills, in mature form, endow one with ''the ability to participate in a variety of groups in a manner that is satisfying for oneself and one's fellow members'' (1970, p. 273). Groups designed for congruency with relative interactional skills then become arenas for developing higher level or more mature skills.

These cited authors (Shannon and Snortum; Fidler; and Mosey) point to the role of the occupational therapy group as an interactional experience which allows for the assessment and enhancement of overall social and functional skills. Other authors have described the use of particular modalities (Rothaus, Hanson, and Cleveland, 1966; Rance and Price, 1973; Angel, 1981) as well as instruction in specific functional skills within a group structure (Hughes and Mullins, 1981).

This discussion, however, will focus on the occupational therapy group as an interactional experience and on the application of such an experience within a short-term psychiatric setting where the overall goals of hospitalization are apt to be diagnostic assessment, reduction of symptomatology, and rapid reintegration into the community. In contrast to long-term outpatient or in-hospital treatment where goals are typically more ambitious in terms of personality reorganization, short-term inpatient treatment is customarily geared toward dealing with the immediate determinants of and precipitants for hospital admission. According to Leeman in his chapter in the recently published *Inpatient Psychiatry—Diagnosis and Treatment* (1983), "this requires evaluating the patient's premorbid environment, assessing the patient's behavior in varied interpersonal situations, and providing opportunities to enhance the patient's responsibility and to restore optimal social functioning" (p. 223).

The short-term unit as a setting for this process tends to have certain characteristic features. The relatively brief period of hospitalization and consequent rapid patient turnover results in a continually fluctuating social situation. Physically the units are usually self-contained within a relatively small space thereby creating the potential of an intensively dynamic environment. Typically, patients have frequent, if not constant, contact throughout the day in terms of sharing a central dayroom, eating in a common dining area, and participating together in various treatment programs. Most clinicians agree that patients in these settings are highly sensitive to events that occur on the unit and fluctuations in its atmosphere. Indeed, the mood of a unit is highly changeable—a volatile situation which erupts into crisis can be followed by a sense of calm resolution within a period of several hours. The patient population itself can also be highly varied in terms of diagnosis and level of function. However, despite this, patients often develop a strong sense of mutual affiliation on the basis of their shared hospitalization. In a further contribution to the dynamics of a short-term unit, individual staff members often serve in a multiplicity of roles which sometimes results in a blurring of these roles. For example, a nurse may function as both a primary therapist who meets psychotherapeutically with a patient and as a charge nurse who administers medication to that same patient.

These, then, are some of the notable features of the short-term psychiatric setting in which an occupational therapy group is developed and its objectives established. One common primary goal is assessment. The occupational therapy group can provide a cost-effective, expeditious and structured means of evaluating an individual's social-interactive skills. Occupational therapists have long identified the potential of their group-oriented programs to provide such assessment. More recently, there has been delineation of the specific aspects of social-interactive functioning that should be included in that assessment. Bloomer and Williams (1982) have described the seven parameters included in their Bay Area Functional Performance Evaluation. These are response to authority figures, verbal communication, psychomotor behavior, independence/dependence, socially appropriate behavior, ability to work with peers and participation in group/program activities. The information yielded by such an assessment is valuable in several ways. For one, it helps to determine what types of consequent treatment experiences might be indicated during hospitalization. Equally important, such assessment can suggest what kinds of treatment might be recommended for outpatient follow-up. In addition, regular participation in an occupational therapy group can provide on-going assessment data that is valuable as an overall index of progress during hospitalization. Obviously, on a short-term unit, assessment and treatment often take place concurrently and one continually impacts on the other.

The group-oriented occupational therapy program is also aimed at providing treatment. On the basis of appropriate evaluation and typically in collaboration with both patient and other staff members, a decision is made as to the advisability of involving the patient in a particular group program. Groups may differ in terms of the modalities used, the content of focus and the expectant level of participant functioning. However, one primary goal is to enhance social-interactive skills in relation to the patient's potential and the demands of the environment to which he/she will return. This overall goal is further delineated in terms of objectives which may include the reinforcement of socially acceptable behavior, the fostering of effective communication skills, the encouragement of self-awareness and self-expression, and the strengthening of interpersonal confidence. King (1978) has postulated that "we could say that occupational therapy consists of structuring the surroundings, materials and especially the demands of the environment in such a way as to call forth a specific adaptive response" (p. 16). A structured occupational therapy group can thus be seen as a setting in which more adaptive interactional skills can be identified and experienced.

In considering the feasibility of pursuing such objectives, it seems necessary to examine their compatability with the setting in which they occur. Leeman (1983) notes that "the essence of inpatient psychiatric treatment . . . is that it occurs in a controlled milieu" (p. 223). Abrams (1969) has defined milieu therapy as "the means of organizing a community treatment environment so that every treatment technique can be specifically utilized to further the patient's aims of controlling symptomatic behaviors and learning appropriate psycho-social skills'' (p. 559). Certainly not all short-term units subscribe to this pure model of milieu therapy; most, however, recognize the environmental aspects of inpatient psychiatry and to varying degrees use the milieu for therapeutic purposes.

There is a strong parallel between the experiential and structured nature of milieu therapy in general and the occupational therapy group in particular. As an occupational therapy group actualizes its own objectives, it also supports the overall therapeutic purpose of inpatient hospitalization. Furthermore, the capacity of the occupational therapy group to provide such catalytic experiences has particular significance in a short-term setting where time is a limited resource and treatment must be goal-oriented. Whether the purpose is to evaluate social-interactive functioning or to foster growth in specific interactional skills, the occupational therapist can actively orchestrate a group program to meet that purpose. Additionally, if comfortably skilled in group dynamics, he/she can personalize and intensify the experience for participant patients and thereby facilitate their active involvement. Therein lies the potential of the occupational therapy group to be an integrative setting in which inpatient experience can be translated into therapeutic growth.

Most therapists who work in short-term units might also add (or perhaps argue!) that the realization of this potential is hampered by the realities that characterize such units. It seems advisable, then, to outline some points to be considered in developing an occupational therapy group as well as to share specific aspects of the author's experience in doing so. Such an outline and discussion follows.

FLEXIBILITY

With as variable a population as typifies a short-term unit, occupational therapists should be prepared to be very flexible in both therapeutic approach and program content. For instance, the focus of a particular group is often determined on a day-to-day basis. Similarly, it is usually impossible to maintain a constant group membership over any extended period of time. Also, a group must be flexible so as to allow for less functional patients while at the same time provide a meaningful experience for those functioning at a higher level. The author, for instance, has developed and co-led a Communication Skills group for one short-term unit. This group met once a week for 1½ hours and averaged 5-6 members. Each group was structured to provide experiences that might increase awareness of communication patterns and encourage exploration of alternative patterns. However, the actual content differed greatly and depended upon the assessment by both the group leadership and other staff members as well as patients themselves as to how the group could be particularly helpful. Job interviewing, conversational skills, assertiveness and self-disclosure were commonly identified as issues to be worked on and role-playing was often used to offer practice in more adaptive ways of handling such situations as they typically arise. Participants were often encouraged to further practice outside the group in hopes of maximizing the overall usefulness of their hospitalization experience.

REALISTIC EXPECTATIONS

Time constraints create a need to be modest in setting goals for a group program. At times, assessment of interactional skills may be the primary goal. At other times, the goal may be to initiate a therapeutic process that will continue after discharge. For instance, based on an individual's participation as an inpatient, he/she might be referred to a group program on an outpatient basis. As an example of adapting expectations, the author had several years of experience being the on-going leader for a traditionally conceived verbal therapy group on a short-term unit. It became increasingly evident that the non-directive leadership and unstructured format that might be appropriate for a long-term outpatient group was not so in a short-term inpatient setting and was perhaps even counter-productive. On this basis, a model of unit-wide Community Meetings was developed for which the author provided primary leadership. These meetings were aimed at encouraging patients to address issues occurring within the community, to exchange perceptions of their day-to-day life together and its relation to life in the community, and to directly resolve conflicts when indicated. Not only did these meetings seem to facilitate the overall functioning of the unit, but they also provided another opportunity for patients to practice social-interactive skills that have relevance to community life outside the hospital.

UNDERSTANDING OF GROUP DYNAMICS
AS REFLECTION OF WARD DYNAMICS

Several authors (Levine, 1980; Kibel, 1981) have suggested the need for the therapist to be sensitive to the connection between the dynamics evident in an inpatient group and the on-going dynamics of the unit as a whole. Not only is this essential to the therapist's interpretation of the group process, but it is also key to the occupational therapy group's existence as an integrated part of the therapeutic whole. Given the previously suggested characteristics of a short-term unit, the interplay of group and ward dynamics may be particularly evident in such a setting. At one time, for instance, the author coordinated a meal preparation program in which patients of a short-term unit were expected to plan and prepare a unit-wide dinner on a weekly basis. The ability of a specified group to work cooperatively toward such a purpose was often affected by the broader dynamics of the unit at the time. An awareness of this was helpful in making the experience optimally therapeutic for those patients involved. A common case in the cooking program was that patients who were dominant figures on the unit at large often took on parallel roles in the meal preparation. This, then, could become an opportunity to allow those patients to share responsibility and to encourage other more passive patients to assert themselves. Sensitivity to the dynamics of the larger population can expedite the purposes of the occupational therapy program as well as make those purposes individually tailored. Given the limited time frame of the short-term unit, both of these aspects are significant.

NEED FOR A SYSTEM PERSPECTIVE

If an occupational therapy group is to survive, let alone succeed, in a short-term unit, its role in the larger system of the unit must be considered. Klein and Kugel (1981) have noted that "it is clear that the social system of the ward—with its norms, expectations and values—plays a particularly important role in determining patient's behavior in group meetings and has a significant impact on therapeutic process" (p. 316). The identity of the group must be congruent or at least compatible with the overall treatment philosophy of the unit. Questions arising from this issue as well as others less directly related should be explored. Is the occupational therapy group sanctioned administratively and supported by other staff? Do the structure and norms of the unit reinforce regular patient attendance? Does the group reflect sensitivity to the value system of its intended participants? It has been the experience of this author, for example, that self-expressive modalities have limited relevance on a short-term unit in a Veterans' Hospital serving a rural population. This might then suggest the advisability of incorporating a task orientation into a particular group. In fact, it was found that a woodworking group that used a modality highly acceptable to a male, work-oriented population was more effective in reinforcing basic interactional skills. Similarly, this kind of group coincided with the values of the larger social system of the institution itself.

NEED FOR EDUCATION AND COLLABORATION

Given the interwoven dynamics and the time limitation that characterize a short-term unit, it seems particularly important that its various staff members work cooperatively. Accordingly, the occupational therapist needs to educate other staff about a particular group and its therapeutic purposes. Inservices as well as opportunities to observe and participate can facilitate staff understanding and support. Issues of professional territorialism can, however, arise and the role of the occupational therapy group may at times need to be coordinated with the efforts of other staff members. Similarly, the author has at times been integrally involved in interdisciplinary treatment programs. This has included, for example, providing co-leadership in a weekly Outward Bound treatment program for selected patients on a short-term unit. Here the role of occupational therapist was to assess the social and functional levels of the participating patients, to suggest appropriate goals for the Outward Bound experience and to facilitate the group dynamics of the experience itself.

These, then, are points that an occupational therapist might consider in developing a group program for a short-term inpatient unit. He/she, however, may still experience frustration with the nature of such a unit. There is the sense of constant beginning and having to start over. The emotional drain resulting from working with individuals in a state of acute dysfunction is considerable and there is little of the satisfaction that may arise from longer-term treatment and the solidified growth that can take place there. Also, it is often difficult to delineate the specific impact of various forms of treatment in a short-term setting. However, the well-conceived and sensitively executed occupational therapy group plays a vital part in the process that allows individuals to regain a sense of their ability to cope and to begin to approach their lives more adaptively. Some find a challenge within these limits—a challenge to their personal ability to adapt just as they challenge that of their patients. Occupational therapy has long proclaimed its ability to assess and enhance the interactional skills of those psychiatric populations served. With careful consideration and some modification, this strong tradition will prevail on the short-term units so prevalent today in psychiatric treatment.

REFERENCES

Abroms, G. M. Defining milieu therapy. *Archives of General Psychiatry,* 1969, *21,* 553-560.

Angel, S. L. The emotion identification group. *American Journal of Occupational Therapy,* 1981, *35,* 256-262.

Bloomer, J., & Williams, S. The Bay Area Functional Performance Evaluation. In B. J. Hemphill (Ed.), *The Evaluative Process in Psychiatric Treatment.* Thorofare, NY: Charles B. Slack, 1981.

Bobis, B., Harrison, R., & Traub, L. Activity group therapy. *American Journal of Occupational Therapy,* 1955, *IX,* 19-21.

Crory, S., Sebastian, V., & Mosey, A. C. Acute short-term treatment in psychiatry. *American Journal of Occupational Therapy,* 1974, *28,* 401-406.

Erickson, R. C. Small-group psychotherapy with patients on a short-stay ward: An opportunity for innovation. *Hospital and Community Psychiatry,* 1983, *32,* 269-272.

Fidler, G. Task-oriented group as a context for treatment. *American Journal of Occupational Therapy,* 1969, *XXIII,* 43-48.

Hughes, P. L., & Mullins, L. *Acute psychiatric care.* Thorofare, NJ: Charles B. Slack, 1981.

Kibel, H. D. A conceptual model for short-term inpatient group psychotherapy. *American Journal of Psychiatry,* 1981, *138,* 74-80.

King, L. J. Toward a science of adaptive responses. *American Journal of Occupational Therapy,* 1978, *32,* 14-22.

Klein, R. H. In patient group psychotherapy: Practical considerations and special problems. *International Journal of Group Psychotherapy,* 1977, *27,* 201-214.

Klein, R. H., & Kugel, B. Inpatient group psychotherapy from a systems perspective: Reflections through a glass darkly. *International Journal of Group Psychotherapy,* 1981, *31,* 311-321.

Leeman, C. P. The therapeutic milieu. In L. I. Sederer (Ed.), *Inpatient Psychiatry: Diagnosis and Treatment.* Baltimore: Williams & Wilkins, 1983.

Levine, H. B. Milieu biopsy: The place of the therapy group on the inpatient ward. *International Journal of Group Psychotherapy,* 1980, *30,* 77-93.

Llorens, L. A. Changing methods in treatment of psychosocial dysfunction. *American Journal of Occupational Therapy,* 1968, *XXII,* 26-29.

Mosey, A. C. The concept and use of developmental groups. *American Journal of Occupational Therapy,* 1970, *xxiv,* 272-275.

Rance, D., & Price, A. Poetry as a group project. *American Journal of Occupational Therapy,* 1973, 27, 252-255.

Rothaus, P., Hanson, P. G., & Cleveland, S. E. Art and group dynamics. *American Journal of Occupational Therapy,* 1966, *20,* 182-187.

Sederer, L. I. (Ed.) *Inpatient psychiatry: Diagnosis and treatment.* Baltimore: Williams & Wilkins, 1983.

Shannon, P. D., & Snortum, J. R. An activity group's role. *American Journal of Occupational Therapy,* 1965, *XIX,* 344-347.

Occupational Therapy for Chronic Pain: A Clinical Application of the Model of Human Occupation

Rebecca Liggan Gusich, MS, OTR

ABSTRACT. The patient with chronic pain presents a dilemma for physical as well as psychiatric health care. Usually coming to the attention of mental health professionals after limited or no successful treatment with medical specialties, these patients present with a variety of factors that disrupt occupational functioning. Occupational therapy is the health profession qualified to analyze occupational function and dysfunction for remedial action of chronic pain behavior. An occupational therapy approach based on the model of human occupation is described. It is proposed as an appropriate treatment strategy for the short-term, acute-care chronic pain patient on a psychiatry service, as part of an interdisciplinary pain program. A discussion of chronic pain, its impact on occupational functioning and the development of an occupational therapy treatment program are presented, along with a case example and implications for further study.

Long before the organized medical and psychosocial sciences became involved with the problems of chronic pain, philosophers and theologians alike had concluded that pain and suffering are invaluable to life itself and not to be avoided (8, 18, 19). Pain as a subjective symptom creates in the sufferer the need for quick relief. Chronic pain, defined as pain that has persisted for more than three months without relief (23, 28), has become "America's hidden epi-

Rebecca Liggan Gusich (Medical College of Virginia—Virginia Commonwealth University, 1978), is Senior Staff Therapist in the Psychiatry Section, Occupational Therapy Department, Medical College of Virginia Hospitals, Box 428, MCV Station, Richmond, Virginia 23298.

The author gratefully acknowledges the assistance of the following persons in the preparation of this manuscript: Gary Kielhofner, Dr. P.H., O.T.R., Florence B. Chichester, M.A., O.T.R., Ann Neville, M.S., O.T.R. and Joseph A. Kwentus, M.D.

demic'' (7). Nearly one-third of America's population has recently reported persistent or recurring chronic pain. It has taken an economic toll of lost wages, medical and related costs and compensation payments, estimated to be as high as 35 to 50 billion dollars per year. Its human toll is thought to involve more than one million American workers on any given day prevented by pain from reporting to work (6, 7, 14).

Chronic pain is a multidimensional problem that erodes the coping capacity of the individual in performance of work, social, familial and leisure roles. Bonica (6, p. vii) states, " . . . it is *not* the underlying pathology but the pain that primarily impairs the patient's carrying out a productive lifestyle." Chronic pain is a stressor of the highest order, as it places excessive and unrelenting demands on the individual to alter environment, roles and habits, and to adopt a pain-centered lifestyle. This altered lifestyle can be viewed as dysfunctional when societal demands and expectations for productivity and playful participation are not met. In addition, the victim's innate urge to explore and master the environment is impaired (16, 25). The model of human occupation addresses occupational dysfunction, thus it is used as the basis for the program described in this paper. While it is recognized that specific pain problems require specific treatment, the purpose of this paper is to relate theoretical concepts of occupational behavior to practice, with the focus on pain *behavior* (regardless of its etiology or manifestation); also, to show the influence of pain behavior on lifestyle, occupational function and dysfunction.

OCCUPATIONAL BEHAVIOR VIEW OF PAIN

The model of human occupation (15, 17) theorizes about the inherent urge to explore and master one's environment which promotes occupational function (16). Conversely, occupational dysfunction is a malfunction in the interaction between the person and environment. A maladaptive cycle results in which there is a disruption in the normal open system cycle of intake, throughput, output and feedback, In addition, there is a breakdown in one or more of the subsystems (volition, habituation and performance).[1] Chronic pain negatively influences every aspect of life, producing an occupational dysfunction.

Volition

The volition subsystem is composed of personal causation, values and interests. In the patient with chronic pain, this subsystem is characterized by decreased self-confidence, loss of normal goals and interests and lack of motivation. Personal causation is eroded by feelings of external control by the pain. The patient in time comes to expect failure because of prior experience with pain's interference with function. The loss of many normal functions and the disruption of normal lifestyles can contribute to low self-esteem in chronic pain patients (2). The patient concerned about perceived limitations may lose belief in skills. For example, a clergyman's wife who had a counseling practice had chronic leg pain. She resolved to decrease her practice because she felt that she would be ineffective with her church members because of her feelings of inadequacy in controlling her own chronic suffering.

Premorbid valued goals begin to deteriorate together with the inherent meaning of most daily activities. The patient views the future as bleak as a result of this obsession with pain. Also, the patient tends to develop new short-term and long-term goals where the focus is on resignation to a life with pain.

A loss of interest in formerly pleasurable activities is a significant component of the description of patients with chronic pain (23). There is a tendency to give up active interests for more sedentary, less active pursuits. The absence of meaning and pleasure in activity should be viewed as a profound loss adding to the patient's suffering. This anhedonia is also a symptom of depression, which often accompanies chronic pain states (5, 23).

Habituation

The habituation subsystem includes internalized roles and habits.[2] It becomes dysfunctional as the individual assumes the role of invalid and develops accompanying habits of dependence. Other roles are also relinquished along with the acquisition of this invalid role. One patient with chronic cancer pain fashioned a habit of dependence when she realized that her pharmacist/husband could continually supply her with addicting pain medications. Such habits become rigidly established as a way of avoiding or diminishing perceived pain.

Performance

The performance subsystem,[3] which incorporates necessary skills for action, is disrupted by the fear that continued performance of skills will intensify the pain. Motor skills are not performed because of actual or perceived limitations. New adaptive skills are not attempted for this same reason, because of interference of psychological, physical or environmental factors.

For the functional individual, information from these subsystems (volition, habituation and performance) is processed from the environment and produces appropriate output action in an adaptive self-maintaining cycle.[4] The maladaptive cycle experienced by the patient with chronic pain is summarized and illustrated in Figure 1. Society reinforces the feedback for this maladaptive cycle as the attention given by significant others perpetuates pain behavior. The emotional components of anxiety, depression, helplessness and hopelessness further cloud the entire occupational performance.

INTERVENTIONS FOR CHRONIC PAIN

There are as many treatment programs for chronic pain as there are disciplines involved in its care (19). For example, physical therapy literature discusses the use of transcutaneous electrical nerve stimulation (TENS), electromyographic (EMG) biofeedback, heat and cold, exercise and other modalities within an operant conditioning approach (24). Flower et al. (12) describe an innovative and cooperative effort between the physical disabilities and psychiatric occupational therapists and members of other disciplines who are involved in a comprehensive program for low back pain. Belar (3), a psychologist, also describes a specific program of stress-management for chronic pain. Her stated focus is correction of maladaptive behaviors and transference of newly-learned coping skills to real situations. Education, relaxation training and skill development are incorporated in her program.

While disciplines have used their own various approaches to remediating pain in relative isolation in the past, more recently the concept of the "Pain Clinic" has evolved. It is a comprehensive, centralized service involving a multidisciplinary, multimodal approach to chronic pain diagnosis and management.[5] The primary objective of pain clinics is to assess the person in a holistic manner,

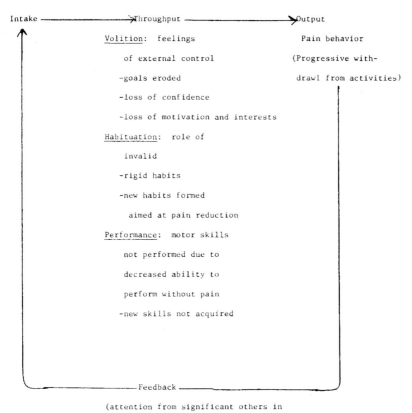

FIGURE 1. Maladaptive Cycle of Chronic Pain Behavior

to identify the influence of the pain behavior on function and to focus on developing ways to counteract the establishment or perpetuation of a pain-centered lifestyle (6). The treatment may include behavioral, social, economic, vocational, cognitive, sensory, physiological, philosophical and/or spiritual approaches. In the context of the interdisciplinary pain program the challenge to occupational therapy is to define its unique contribution to the care of the pain patient.

THE IN-PATIENT PAIN TREATMENT PROGRAM

The occupational therapy program described in this paper is part of the In-patient Pain Treatment Program, which is an individualized multidisciplinary service of the Division of Consultation/Liaison Psychiatry at the Medical College of Virginia Hospital. As with many other pain programs, there is a team approach, consisting of a psychiatrist (along with resident physician and/or rotating medical students), as well as the adjunctive services of nursing, social work, psychology, pharmacology, chaplain program, physical therapy and occupational therapy. The primary goal of the program is to change the patient's role from that of being a passive recipient of attention via pain behavior to becoming an active participant in more adaptive functioning.

Physicians assess the location of the pain, etiology and the possibility of drug dependence due to the initial pain. Nursing staff members perform many functions related to 24-hour management of pain complaints and act as interpreters and empathic supporters of the patient's daily interactions with pain. The social worker may be involved as the liaison between the hospital management of the patient and the family by keeping them informed of the patient's status. The social worker also counsels family members to help them learn to support the patient's more adaptive behavior post-discharge. The psychologist develops behavioral programs and provides objective data regarding pain personality profiles through standardized tests. The pharmacologist may be called upon to lend expertise in medication-weaning. The chaplain may provide the spiritual guidance to the patient as well as to the team. The physical therapist offers the patient a variety of physical modalities and exercise for subjective and objective relief of the pain. In the context of these interdisciplinary services occupational therapy offers a program aimed at enhancing the everyday occupational behavior of patients.

OCCUPATIONAL THERAPY PROGRAM: ASSESSMENT AND INTERVENTION

The psychiatric occupational therapy program for chronic pain at the Medical College of Virginia Hospital (MCVH) is also multimodal. It uses existing treatment groups designed to explore and enhance leisure skills, homemaking skills, grooming skills, financial skills, job skills and social skills, as appropriate. Stress management instruction and assertiveness training are also a major part of the program. The occupational therapy rationale for stress management comes from the recognition that chronic pain is a major negative stressor. As Addison states (1, p. 12), " . . . the ability of patients to cope with their pain is largely a function of ability to cope with other stressors prior to onset of pain." In terms of the model of human occupation, negative or excessive stress is seen as eroding the adaptive open system cycle and negatively impacting the subsystems as described earlier. Stress management is therefore viewed as an appropriate approach for restoring a normal cycle of healthy occupational behavior. Along with training the person in developing coping skills specifically for stress management, the occupational therapy program focuses on more practical lifestyle changes that would reduce stress. This may include time management and balance of work/play/rest and sleep. Further, restoration of volition, especially personal causation, is the cornerstone of treatment since choices for lifestyle change must proceed from this subsystem.

Assessment Process

Each patient referred to occupational therapy is given an individualized interview/evaluation to determine both functional level and deficits. A self-assessment questionnaire is given, as appropriate, to assess general awareness, cognitive and organizational abilities, as well as the patient's insight into deficits in life skills functioning (i.e., job, homemaking, financial, leisure, grooming or social). Preliminary goals and the patient's motivation are determined by the therapist and the patient together based on assessment data. Also, appropriate treatment groups are suggested, agreed upon and/or encouraged.

The individualized chronic pain treatment program involves further assessment in specific occupational areas. Table I illustrates the assessment tools used, as well as possible treatment goals accompanying occupational dysfunction in each subsystem. These instruments address the various aspects of the subsystems of volition, habituation and performance previously described and pertinent to the treatment of chronic pain patients. Assessments may include the Social Readjustment Rating Scale (13), the Life Goals Inventory (9), the Internal-External Locus of Control Scale (26), a revised Interest Checklist (27), the Role Checklist (20) and an adapted Activi-

Table I

Assessment Tools Used as Part of Occupational Therapy Pain Treatment Program

Subsystem	Pain-related occupational dysfunction	Assessment tool	Occupational therapy treatment
Volition			
Personal causation	-loss of self-confidence -external view of pain control	- I-E Scale	-restore self-confidence -adopt view of internal control
Valued goals	-loss of normal goals -bleak view of future with pain	- Life Goals Inventory	-identify new goals
Interests	-loss of interests due to perceived or actual pain	- Interest Checklist	-adopt new interests as substitute for ones given up
Habituation			
Internalized roles	-possible reduction or redistribution of roles -acquisition of invalid role	- Role Checklist	-identify needs and abilities for role performance -adapt roles through re-education

Table 1 (continued)

Subsystem	Pain-related occupational dysfunction	Assessment tool	Occupational therapy treatment
Habits	-increased dependence on others -imbalance of lifestyle with more idle time or pain-centered time -rigidity of habits	-Self-Assessment Questionnaire -Activity Questionnaire	-help patient to develop new habits to decrease stress -re-education regarding ideas for low-stress living and working
Performance Skills	-loss of work opportunities -limitations due to pain -lack of exploration of new skill areas -reduction of social skills or assertiveness -decreased coping skills	-Life Skills Assessment with craft activity or other task -Self-Assessment Questionnaire -Social Readjustment Rating Scale	-instruction in relaxation techniques to gain mastery over pain -explore alternative vocational or leisure pursuits -assertiveness training -coping strategies for stress

ty Questionnaire (21). Each patient is asked to complete these assessments independently and to return them to the therapist for scoring and interpretation. If appropriate, observational data are also collected during the patient's participation in various performance groups (job skills or leisure skills craft groups, for example). All of these assessment data are summarized and interpreted to the patient by the therapist.

Treatment Process

The treatment process centers around alteration of maladaptive occupational behavior due to the stress of chronic pain through the patient's understanding of how chronic pain has caused significant occupational lifestyle changes. The groundwork is laid once the climate of patient awareness is created, fostering the development of adaptive coping skills or new habits. Setting of realistic expectations is essential and the patient is encouraged to create a list of long-term and short-term goals for later discussion. Educational material is provided regarding ideas for low-stress living in areas of home, work and leisure functioning. This educational material is designed to help restore a sense of personal causation as well as goals, interests, roles, habits and skills. It is used in discussion as well as in written plans for future use by the patient. If not already taught by other staff, relaxation training techniques such as Benson's "Relaxation Response" (4) or progressive muscle relaxation are taught, along with deep-breathing techniques for stress-control to develop skills for mastery of stressful pain. Assertiveness training, especially learning to respond to persuasion (i.e., "saying no") and assertive expression of feelings may be incorporated. It has been shown that many patients with chronic pain syndrome have non-assertive or passive/aggressive communication styles (24).

Individual treatment sessions may last from an average of thirty minutes to one hour, depending on the topic and tolerance of the patient. They are primarily discussion and guidance format, although the patient plays an active role in developing a repertoire of coping skills. A variety of areas are discussed, all progressing toward predetermined goals. They include stress on the job, coping with family expectations, resolving feelings about need to decrease activity, increase activity or develop adaptive activities, preparing for return to work or a new job, peer relations, etc. The patient's changing roles, interests and skills are emphasized and practiced in role-play situations. Personal causation and self-responsibility are reinforced with each session. Healthy occupational functioning is thus the goal for the program, and may be demonstrated by therapeutic passes for the patient with and without escorts as appropriate, so that the patient may prove his or her own control over maladaptive pain behavior.

The following case example is presented as illustration of this assessment and treatment approach.

Case Description

Dan is a 39-year-old white married male with a history of injury to the lower thoracic spine due to a fall at home six years prior to his current hospitalization on the in-patient psychiatric unit. Another spinal injury to the same area occurred approximately one year after the initial trauma. After extensive evaluations by orthopedic and neuorological specialists with only temporary relief from the pain, Dan consented to psychological and psychiatric attempts at management. On psychological testing, he was shown to have some deficits in new learning that decreased his memory and increased his anxiety. A non-assertive communication style was also noted. Medical management was accomplished through treatment with mild muscle relaxants along with supportive psychotherapy and TENS from physical therapy. He also participated in writing a pain diary with assistance from the nursing staff. The following occupational therapy intervention took place.

On assessment, Dan was noted to have problems related to work (stressful performance and strained relations with boss), decreased motivation for leisure interests and an acknowledged lack of assertiveness, as well as inability to cope with the stress of his back pain. Further assessments given (Buhler Life Goals Inventory, Holmes and Rahe Social Readjustment Rating Scale, Rotter Internal-External Locus of Control Scale, Oakley Role Checklist and Scaffa revised Interest Checklist) revealed information regarding his occupational dysfunction. Table II summarizes Dan's occupational strengths and weaknesses, in a manner similar to that described by Cubie and Kaplan (11). Although Dan felt responsible for directing most events in his life, he expressed the feeling that pain controlled his lifestyle, limiting every move and increasing stress. He was acutely aware of recent stressful life events and the consequent interests and roles given up, including leisure pursuits and some family activities. His chronic disability contributed to his depressed

Table II

Case Summary: Dan

Introductory data: 39 y.o.m., dx chronic pain, depression

Tools used: Social Readjustment Rating Scale, revised Interest Checklist, Life Goals Inventory,
Role Checklist, I-E Locus of Control Scale, Self-Assessment Questionnaire.

Analysis	Degree of problem for patient	Comments	Occupational therapy treatment
Personal causation	-mild dysfunction	-patient aware of need to develop internal control but unable	-empathic feedback and support and opportunity for development of coping skills
Valued goals	-moderate dysfunction	-anger/guilt about lack of goal achievement	-identification of realistic goals
Interests	-mod./severe dysf.	-patient began to perceive interests as "chores"	-exploration of new interests
Internalized roles	-moderate dysfunction	-limited currently by pain and not expressed	-development of congruent role expectations
Habits	-moderate dysfunction	-limited and rigid	-alteration through practice
Skills	-mild dysfunction	-adequate performance of work though limited coping skills	-increase coping skills -relaxation training -assertiveness training

70

mood and severely limited his desired roles of breadwinner and strong family figure.

Dan was highly motivated for change and participated readily in the occupational therapy treatment program of individual lifestyle restructuring which incorporated stress-management and assertiveness training. The primary focus was a limited number of sessions (approximately 30-45 minutes each) with the use of patient education materials and verbal exploration of stressors, coping strategies, relaxation exercises and assertiveness information and practice.

Patient education materials included a bibliography with specific suggestions for his particular pain dysfunction. After identification of stressors from the assessment, Dan used his list to focus on what could be altered in the future or at least anticipated. Coping strategies for Dan included habit change (prioritizing and time management), pursuit of new leisure interests (individual, social and with family), utilization of his sense of humor in positive thinking and planning and the development of a sense of self-control. He participated in deep-breathing exercises and previously-learned progressive muscle relaxation via cassette tapes. Assertiveness information for Dan included "saying no" without feeling guilty (using practice exercises from several books from his bibliography) and assertiveness to a superior in the job setting. General problem-solving skills were taught and reinforced when pain interfered with decision-making. Dan expressed interest in maintaining new skills post-discharge. He has continued to supply periodic progress reports to occupational therapy via his out-patient psychiatrist, and expressed positive results and attempts to maintain healthy occupational functioning.

SUMMARY AND IMPLICATIONS FOR FURTHER STUDY

Rationale for the use of the model of human occupation for treatment of chronic pain patients seen on the in-patient psychiatry service has been presented. A description of the patient with chronic pain and consequent dysfunction in aspects of human occupation has been discussed as a means of translating theoretical concepts into practical application. The application of these concepts has been demonstrated in a case example.

Further substantive data through development of quantitative measurements to assess treatment programs would yield results as to the efficacy of the program. Also of value would be studies of the different personality factors which may influence the success of this treatment program. Specific areas, such as vocational assessment or homemaking ability, may be further studied as they relate to the dysfunction created by chronic pain. The magnitude and potential for the problem must be addressed; as S. B. Chayatte (10, p. 116) relates, from personal experience, " . . . when a person ceases to function, to be productive, we all lose something. We must recycle our disabled workers. If each of us grows dependent on someone else, who will be left to support us all?''

REFERENCES

1. Addison, R. G. Treatment of chronic pain: the Center for Pain Studies, Rehabilitation Institute of Chicago. In Ng, L.K.Y., ed. *New approaches to treatment of chronic pain.* Rockville, Md.: National Institute on Drug Abuse, 1981.

2. Armentrout, D. P. The impact of chronic pain on the self-concept. *Journal of Clinical Psychology,* 1979, 35(3), 517-521.

3. Belar, C. D. Stress management of chronic pain. *Journal of the Florida Medical Association,* 1980, 65(5), 487-490.

4. Benson, H. *The relaxation response.* New York: William Morrow & Co., Inc., 1975.

5. Black. R. G. Clinical syndrome of chronic pain. In Ng, L.K.Y., and Bonica, J. J., eds. *Pain, discomfort, and humanitarian care.* New York: Elsevier/N. Holland, 1980.

6. Bonica, J. J. Preface. In Ng, L.K.Y., ed. *New approaches to treatment of chronic pain.* Rockville, Md.: National Institute on Drug Abuse, 1981.

7. Brena, S. F., ed., Introduction. In *Chronic pain: America's hidden epidemic.* New York: Atheneum/SMI, 1978.

8. Brena, S. F. Lessons from the great religions. In Brena, S. F., ed. *Chronic pain: America's hidden epidemic.* New York: Atheneum/SMI, 1978.

9. Buhler, C. Life goals inventory (available for use from G. Kielhofner, M.A., O.T.R., Dr.P.H. Department of Occupational Therapy, Medical College of Virginia, Richmond, Va. 23298).

10. Chayette, S. B. A personal commitment to health may lead to a lifestyle relatively pain-free. In Brena, S. F. *Chronic pain: America's hidden epidemic.* New York: Atheneum/SMI, 1978.

11. Cubie, S. and Kaplan, K. A case analysis method for the model of human occupation. *American Journal of Occupational Therapy,* 1982, 36(10), 645-656.

12. Flower, A., Naxon, E., Jones, R., Mooney, V. An occupational therapy program for chronic back pain. *American Journal of Occupational Therapy,* 1981, 35(4), 243-248.

13. Holmes, T. H. and Rahe, R. H. The social readjustment rating scale. *Journal of Psychosomatic Reserach,* 1967, 11(8), 213-218.

14. Jacobs, D. D. Holistic strategies in the management of chronic pain. In McGuigan, F., Sime, W., and Wallace, J., eds. *Stress and tension control.* New York: Plenum Press, 1980.

15. Kielhofner, G. A model of human occupation, part 3: benign and vicious cycles. *American Journal of Occupational Therapy,* 1980, 34(11), 731-737.

16. Kielhofner, G. Occupational function and dysfunction. Manuscript for publication in

Kielhofner, G., ed. *A model of human occupation: theory and application,* (in press, Williams & Wilkins).

17. Kielhofner, G. and Burke, J. A model of human occupation, part 1: conceptual framework and content. *American Journal of Occupational Therapy,* 1980, 34(9), 572-581.

18. Lewis, C. S. *The problem of pain.* New York: Macmillan, 1943.

19. Melzack, R. *The puzzle of pain.* New York: Basic Books, 1973.

20. Oakley, F. Role checklist. Unpublished master's project, Department of Occupational Therapy, Medical College of Virginia 23298, 1982.

21. Occupational Therapy Department. Activity Questionnaire. Unpublished manuscript, adapted from N. Riopel's Occupational Questionnaire, 1982, NIH Clinical Center, Bethesda, Md. 20205.

22. Pelletier, K. *Mind as healer, mind as slayer.* New York: Delacorte Press, 1977.

23. *Report of the panel on pain to the National Advisory Neurological and Communicative Disorders and Stroke Council,* U.S. Department HEW, Washington, D.C., 1979.

24. Roesch, R. and Ulrich, D. Physical therapy management in the treatment of chronic pain. *Physical Therapy,* 1980, 60(1), 53-57.

25. Rogers, J. Order and disorder in medicine and occupational therapy. *American Journal of Occupational Therapy,* 1982, 36(1), 29-35.

26. Rotter, J. Generalized expectancies for internal vs. external control of reinforcement. *Psychological Monographs,* 1966, 80, 1-28.

27. Scaffa, M. Revised interest checklist. Unpublished master's project, Department of Occupational Therapy, Medical College of Virginia, Richmond, Virginia 23298, 1981.

28. Smoller, B. and Schulman, B. Chronic pain: prevention through early intervention. *Occupational Health and Safety,* 1981, 50(3), 14-21.

FOOTNOTES

1. See G. Kielhofner and J. Burke, A model of human occupation, part 1: conceptual framework and content. *American Journal of Occupational Therapy,* 1980, 34(9), 572-581.

2. See Footnote 1.

3. See Footnote 1.

4. See Footnote 1.

5. See L.K.Y. Ng, ed. *New approaches to treatment of chronic pain, a review of multidisciplinary pain clinics and pain centers.* Rockville, Maryland: National Institute on Drug Abuse, 1981.

Short-Term Hospital Treatment
of the Acute Schizophrenic Episode

Boaz Harris, MD

Some third-party payors tell us that the median period of hospitalization for an acute schizophrenic episode should be twenty-one to twenty-three days. Although there is no reason for us to modify our psychiatric care of the patient to suit third-party carriers, a need exists not only to help control the increasing costs of hospital treatment but also to relieve the acute suffering of both the patient and the patient's family when an acute schizophrenic episode—the initial schizophrenic episode or an acute exacerbation of the illness—occurs.

Because the initial referral is often made by the family physician, there is considerable value in taking a brief history of the patient from the physician and also inquiring about the incidence of similar illness in the family. The admissions are generally emergencies and thus often cannot be scheduled at a time convenient for the psychiatrist or for the hospital staff.

If at all possible, the physician should be available to receive the patient and the family in his office if the physician is hospital-based. If the physician has immediate commitments to other patients, one staff member should act as the leader and introduce him or herself. There is some merit in having both a male and a female staff member meet the patient on admission in that a given patient may react more constructively to a staff member of one or the other sex. In general, one should not even offer a handshake in that the acutely disturbed schizophrenic patient may perceive this as an hostile act or

Dr. Harris is medical director of Peachford Hospital, and assistant clinical professor of psychiatry at Emory University, in Atlanta Georgia.

This article was originally published in the National Association of Private Psychiatric Hospitals Journal, Volume 10, Number 4, and is reprinted here with the permission of the publisher.

sexual advance. If the patient, however, offers to shake hands, then one staff member should shake hands with the patient.

The initial reception is quite important to the patient and the patient's family: if the staff is calm and not frightened by the patient's hyperactivity, disorganization, and aggressive behavior, the patient will often temporarily organize a little better and be cooperative in voluntary hospitalization. Moreover, the presence of a well-trained, calm staff often reassures the family; and, as the family's anxiety diminishes, the patient will often show better control.

Admission should be accomplished quite rapidly and the patient's rights should be respected and read to the patient. Our procedure requires that the patient know his rights and sign acknowledgement that he has been advised of his rights at the time of hospitalization. If the patient is highly disturbed and is in danger of being of immediate harm to himself or others or is unable to care for his bodily needs and refuses to enter the hospital voluntarily, then prompt lawful commitment procedures should be instituted.

If the physician is not immediately available, one of the staff members of the therapeutic community to which the patient is assigned takes a history from the patient; a second staff member may take a history from the family. A nursing assessment is always done immediately upon admission. If the schedule of the social service department permits, a detailed social history is taken that day. The social history is rarely delayed more than two days after admission.

If the patient appears to be acutely combative or on the verge of being physically resistive, the patient should be gently approached by the staff member in charge. It is important that the staff members not show fear and that additional staff—who may be needed to restrain the patient—be at a reasonable distance from the patient so that the patient does not have the feeling that he is in imminent danger of being physically overwhelmed.

If the staff member acting as the leader makes the approach and tries to structure the patient with the patient becoming immediately resistive, then the staff must act rapidly to restrain the patient. Once the decision to physically restrain the patient is made, the staff should act quickly with the patient being restrained as rapidly and as safely as possible. It is generally unwise to defer acting once the decision has been made that the patient requires restraint because the patient will sense the threat and will often find a way of using furniture or a corner of a room to defend himself from what he sees as an unreasonable attack. Our procedure permits the patient to be promptly integrated into his or her therapeutic community if feasible; and, generally the patient will be immediately included in all activities after the admitting procedures and the nursing assessment are accomplished.

DEVELOPING A MULTIDISCIPLINARY TREATMENT PLAN

As soon as the social service intake history is done a treatment plan is developed. The physician is primarily responsible for the treatment plan and is joined by the registered nurse in charge of the therapeutic community and all of the nursing staff and mental health assistants in that community. The social workers, recreational therapist, occupational therapist, art therapist, music therapist, and dance therapist also contribute to the overall multidisciplinary treatment plan. In our hospital it is the custom for physicians to see their acutely schizophrenic patients on a daily basis until they stabilize and then reduce the frequency of visits to three to six times weekly.

WORKING WITH THE FAMILY

It is not unusual for the family to be almost as disturbed as the patient or for one or more of the family members to be suffering from this illness to some degree. It is important, therefore, that the social service department and the acutely disturbed family meet as rapidly as possible. The social worker will give some general information to the family about the hospital and the treatment program. The role of the family in providing a psychosocial history that includes a detailed family history and developmental history of the patient will be explained.

The social worker will also deal with the family's immediate guilt and grief in this catastrophic situation: it will be explained to the family that although the circumstances are difficult it is not an unusual experience for a family to go through this type of crisis; the social worker will deal with their feeling of panic and terror that the patient will never get better. Their guilt about not perceiving the illness earlier or bringing the patient to psychiatric care at an earlier time will be discussed. This is the beginning point with the family.

After the psychosocial history is obtained, a decision will be made at the multidisciplinary treatment planning conference about involving the family in family therapy and perhaps in multiple family therapy. If they are involved in family therapy—regrettably some families are reluctant to become involved, having labeled the hospitalized member of the family "the crazy one"—they will also be helped to learn something about schizophrenic behavior. The fear on the part of parents and siblings that the disease is hereditary will be discussed. As the patient progresses, plans for aftercare will be developed. This may include home care, continuing intensive psychotherapy, continuing medication, partial hospitalization or a day patient program. The family's need to find magical cures such as the use of megavitamins, trace minerals, and dialysis will have to be resolved.

An effort is made to reinforce the family's coping mechanisms; and, if the family is substantially disturbed—which is a frequent occurrence—continuing family therapy will be recommended. If another family member is identified as having substantial psychiatric problems, individual therapy will be arranged.

There is considerable merit in having a social worker deal with the family because this permits the psychiatrist to focus entirely on the patient except for multidisciplinary treatment planning conferences and some casework supervision. Very often the patient feels persecuted by the family and it becomes quite imperative that the patient's therapeutic alliance with his psychiatrist be honored and strengthened.

Sometimes a family totally refuses to participate in family therapy, identifying the patient as the crazy one and refusing to do anything other than provide insurance forms and pay the balance of the hospital and physician's bill. In these instances it is important that the patient recognize that the psychiatrist and social worker have made a firm recommendation for the family to have continuing treatment and that the patient understand that his psychiatrist has a clear perception of the general disruption in the family.

ESTABLISHING TRUST

Establishing a warm, trusting relationship between the psychiatrist and the acutely ill schizophrenic patient is essential. The patient must be oriented to reality; the psychotic symptoms must be dealt with; the patient's concept of the world as a rejectomat must be managed. The purpose of the hospitalization is to help the patient reestablish some trust both in himself and others to help him on the road toward establishing healthful, interpersonal relationships.

If there is an early constructive relationship between the psychiatrist and the patient, it facilitates the patient's staying for continuing therapy with a more positive attitude while encouraging the patient to cooperate in milieu therapy and psychotherapy. With a good initial relationship the patient will be much more cooperative in taking his medication, participating in the various therapies, and also participating in the aftercare planning.

INTRODUCING THE PATIENT INTO THE MILIEU

In approaching the acutely psychotic patient it is tremendously important that the psychiatrist not show fear or anxiety. The patient already sees himself as a bad person, rejected by parent figures and humanity in general. We slowly, gently, and in a caring manner introduce the patient into the milieu. We will often introduce the patient to an empathetic patient who is adjusting reasonably well. We constantly reorient the schizophrenic patient for time, place and person, and reality in general. We give much structure and much support.

Sometimes we will listen to the delusional material and will ask the patient to explain what the delusional material means. We will share their feelings, accept the part that is real and help them understand the part that is not real. We make them feel comfortable in sharing and help them establish a sense of trust.

We are heavily staffed at all times because we want staff members readily available to reassure the patients that we are keeping them safe, that we care about them, and that we will not let them harm themselves. We accept their anger and their rage with a minimum of fear; but, we are alert to the fact that the highly disturbed schizophrenic can become precipitously violent. It takes a considerable period of time—even with the help of modern neuroleptics—to wean them back to reality. At the same time we are introducing the patient into the milieu, we are also involving the family in family therapy although it may not be feasible to include the patient in family therapy until the patient has been hospitalized for several weeks. Again, I must comment that there are occasions when it is almost as difficult to orient the family to reality as it is to orient the patient to reality.

A NEED FOR SPACE AND DISTANCE

Too much closeness is frightening to the schizophrenic patient. The patient can easily misinterpret caring and structuring for a hostile threat or a sexual approach. There are occasions where even the large size of a male staff member may be threatening. Although our experience shows that a male schizophrenic often can be structured more easily by female staff members than male staff members, some male schizophrenics will see a small, gentle, caring female staff member as much more threatening than a large, strong, firm male staff member. It is imperative that the staff be aware of where the patient is emotionally at any given time. The staff must not only set limits in their approaches but also must be gentle, consistent, caring, and firm—not judgmental or overly authoritative.

THE THERAPEUTIC COMMUNITY

Our nursing units are somewhat larger than we might desire, and we thus divide each community. The psychiatric service is supervised by a service director who takes responsibility for the milieu and for the operation of the therapeutic communities. We have the usual structure of nursing supervisors; but, in addition to this, each therapeutic community has a registered nurse as team leader and is staffed with registered nurses, licensed practical nurses, and mental health assistants.

The team is supported by an individual social worker for each therapeutic community and thus we are able to emphasize family therapy and aftercare. The various activities therapists support the therapeutic communities. Each community moves as a group to each activity and the community itself is involved as a unit in group therapy with a leader and a co-leader.

We are aware that many schizophrenics cannot tolerate our full schedule of activities and that they are extremely sensitive to multiple external stimuli. We will make exceptions in our intensive activities program for highly disturbed schizophrenics but only if the psychiatrist in charge writes an order to reduce the frequency of activities. We emphasize the value of each patient trying to relate to all members of the community and all of the staff that form part of his therapeutic community.

Unfortunately, many patients who have identified themselves or have been identified as "bad" people see the levels system as a reward and punishment system. We, therefore, utilize a levels system in a constructive therapeutic manner:

- initially when a patient is admitted he is placed on a "unit" status, which means that he moves about the hospital with his therapeutic community—with a staff member always present to structure him and the group;
- when weekly levels meetings are held, including all patients and the multidisciplinary staff, the patient may be moved to the next level, "hospital with buddy." This gives the patient a feeling of more independence but it also places him with another patient so that they can both be of value in orienting one another to time, responsibility, and reality;
- our next level is "hospital" status in which the patient may have freedom of the hospital but may not miss any scheduled activities;
- when the patient becomes distinctly better organized he is given "grounds" privileges, which allow him the freedom of the hospital and campus;
- the next level is an "off grounds" level that permits the patient to start to resume outside responsibilities, including job and school; and,
- we can gradually place some patients on a partial hospitalization schedule.

SECLUSION

We avoid seclusion wherever possible; but, when a patient becomes dangerous to himself or others, seclusion may be indicated. As soon as the patient is properly and legally admitted to the hospital the patient may, on orders of the admitting physician, be removed to a seclusion room and properly restrained. It is my custom to institute treatment promptly on highly disturbed patients using a major tranquilizer. The patient's responses are recorded every fifteen minutes and the blood pressure is monitored hourly.

As soon as the patient is in good control the injectable medication is discontinued and concentrate in similar dosage is continued on an hourly basis as needed for severe agitation; and, when the patient is in good control the dosage is modified to a qid daily dose. The purpose of using the concentrate rather than the tablets is because of the tendency of many schizophrenic patients, particularly those with substantial paranoid ideation, to cheek the medication and dispose of it. During the period of supervision in the seclusion room the patient's fluids are monitored very closely and the patient is freely offered semisolid and solid foods that may appeal to him.

Only staff who are comfortable in the presence of disturbed schizophrenic patients are permitted to deal with the patient. As a hospital-based psychiatrist, my custom is to see the patient several times daily for brief periods during the acute episode. Needless to say, during this time visitors are not permitted. As soon as the patient is able to leave the seclusion area he is integrated into the program of his assigned therapeutic community. Patients who have a high potential for elopement or suicide are not permitted to leave the unit but do participate in all of the activities of their therapeutic community.

We will structure a highly disturbed patient with a tight one-to-one so that a staff member is with the patient at all times. As he becomes more organized he will be placed on loose one-to-one and will be checked by a staff member at fifteen minute intervals. Some patients do very well if they keep their own structure sheet that helps orient them to time, place, and reality. We will require a patient on a structure sheet to check in with a staff member every fifteen or thirty minutes depending on the patient's needs.

If a patient begins to become disturbed and cannot verbally ventilate his feelings in a constructive manner, we will structure the patient to a quiet room. We orient many of our very explosive patients toward asking for time-out so that if they feel they cannot deal with too many external stimuli and feel they are becoming explosive they can request a short period of time in their own room or in a quiet room.

PATIENT GOVERNMENT

Within the therapeutic community, patient government provides some type of order and organization to the psychotic patient and the community. It clarifies roles, helps resolve grievances, and brings patients and staff together. It gives the schizophrenic patient a sense of partial control at a time when he is struggling with control issues. It helps him organize around specific goals and builds self-esteem.

The schizophrenic patient can model himself on the officers of the community and the committee chairmen who have learned to organize better and take responsibility. Community meetings also provide some reasonable degree of closeness without excessive closeness, which is so threatening to many schizophrenics. It is the custom in our hospital for each patient to have an interpersonal relationship (IPR) with a staff member during the day shift and during the evening shift. In dealing with the patient, one avoids talking directly about him. It is best to begin the relationship by talking about something reasonably concrete and objective, perhaps sports, music, gardening, school, or job. It is important to let him ventilate how he feels about the hospital and the therapeutic community.

He will perceive the therapeutic community as a family and will often assume that he has been singled out as the bad, crazy person in the therapeutic community just as he has been identified as the bad, crazy person in the family. It is very important that all members of the staff be consistent and that their report and nursing notes be used to communicate any special problems or changes in the approach to the patient. Although it is not unusual for a patient to single out one staff member consistently for IPRs, it is best if the patient gradually learns to share feelings and seek acceptance from multiple staff members on a one-to-one basis.

The staff should encourage the individual patient to share his feelings with his psychiatrist. The patient will generally see the psychiatrist as an omnipotent, judgmental, controlling individual who is similar to one or both of his parents. It is, therefore, important that the patient be oriented to the fact that his psychiatrist is his doctor who cares about him and is interested in treating him and helping him make a reasonably good adjustment outside the hospital setting.

It is important that there be close communication between the psychiatrist and the staff treating the individual patient. The psychiatrist should have weekly rounds with the staff and participate very actively in the multidisciplinary treatment plan as well as periodic modifications of the plan.

Progress notes should be very informative and any modification in the treatment plan should be documented in the progress notes in order that staff members on all three shifts, the activities staff, and the social services department be aware of any changes in the approach to the patient. When a crisis arises, special meetings should be held and very often a five minute conference with the staff at report will resolve serious treatment problems concerning a highly disturbed patient.

GROUP THERAPY

Group therapy is extremely threatening to the majority of schizophrenics. They may perceive the group as being their own family where they feel they have been judged, attacked, and rejected. Many disturbed schizophrenics even fear the closing of the door. We will close the door but will never lock it. We make it clear to a highly disturbed patient that he can ask to be excused from the group if he is too frightened by the closeness and the subject matter. We are tolerant of patients moving about during group if it is extremely difficult for them to sit still for a sixty minute period. If a patient has an intense fear of losing control, we will structure him out of the group therapy room or permit him to take the initiative to leave.

Because he has usually been raised in an environment in which one or both parents are excessively preoccupied with what other people might think about the family, the patient is quite fearful that the rest of the group will be judgmental. Other patients in the group can often reinforce and support realistic interpretations of the patient and accept the patient's valid feelings. The inappropriate behavior, rambling, and blocking of the highly disturbed schizophrenic patient can often greatly stress the group leader and the group co-leader. In our experience group therapy is more profitable to the schizophrenic patient if an IPR can follow group therapy to help orient the patient to what was real and what was not real.

Many schizophrenics will use muteness to create distance and will occasionally make hostile, sarcastic, attacking comments to keep people from getting close to them. The more disturbed schizophrenic who will act, laugh, and talk inappropriately frequently disrupts the group but over a period of time will become more responsive to structure from the group, the group leader, and the group co-leader. We strive for the patient to relate to all members of the group; but, realistically in short-term hospitalization, the patient rarely can get to the point at which he can feel safe with every member of the group.

ELECTROSHOCK THERAPY

Electroshock therapy no longer plays a significant role in the treatment of the acute schizophrenic episode. Some catatonic patients will not respond to injectable neuroleptics and thus there is little choice other than to utilize electroshock therapy to interrupt the catatonic episode. A rare paranoid schizophrenic will not respond to high dosages of neuroleptics either singly or in combination. If medication, milieu therapy, and individual psychotherapy prove to be of no value in the highly disturbed patient—particularly if there is extreme hyperactivity and difficulty in maintaining nutrition—electroshock therapy may then be indicated.

ACTIVITIES THERAPIES

We utilize the activities therapies intensively as part of a totally integrated multidisciplinary therapeutic approach:

□ at its most basic level, occupational therapy can be utilized to enable a patient to make concrete touch with reality. It can help the patient to organize, improve his memory, and improve his attention span. Occupational therapy projects can raise self-esteem and help the patient perceive what he can achieve in a realistic manner. During occupational therapy we favor some interaction between the patient and his peer group, establishing interpersonal contact while also being involved in a realistic activity;

□ the mind and the body go hand in hand and very often when the patient becomes psychologically withdrawn the body will also withdraw. Often when the body becomes activated the mind will become more integrated with the body. Recreational therapy, therefore, plays an important role in our program and is mandatory for all patients. As soon as the patient is integrated into his therapeutic community one of our recreational therapists will introduce himself to the patient and will discuss our philosophy of recreational therapy as well as explore the patient's interests in various types of recreational activity.

In some recreational activities, which are limited to the unit, the patient will be involved in very quiet group activities and games. Additionally, although patients are told that they do not have to be highly skilled athletes to participate and enjoy our various athletic activities, all patients are encouraged to participate in a very active athletic program. As the patient participates in team recreational activities, he is oriented to reality, begins to socialize, learns to interact with other team members, and has a useful and constructive outlet for his anger. With improved coordination and with the reactivation of old skills or the learning of new skills, the patient's self-image improves.

We have had schizophrenic patients who will constantly hallucinate while alone in their rooms; but, when becoming active in recreational therapy with other patients, they somehow will come together, focus on the activity, and be able to relate constructively to other individuals;

□ most schizophrenics can partially organize visually even if they do not seem to be able to organize verbally. They can draw their fears and their hallucinations and begin to look at them separately as something outside of themselves. They can focus on the external far better than on the internal. It is possible to point out significant features in their art work and begin to discuss and share them with the patients.

For many schizophrenics it is far easier to comment on their drawings than to talk about their intimate feelings in individual or group psychotherapy. For them, the drawings are something real. Patients who are very schizophrenic often do not understand what is real within them or even what is or is not real about their bodies. It is interesting, therefore, to see a schizophrenic patient draw himself as a fragmented human being and discuss the fragmentation. However, if you would ask this patient how he feels he would most probably say "fine";

□ dance therapy can be of considerable value even in the short-term treatment of the schizophrenic patient. Until the patient starts to organize, however, the patient must be in a position to be structured and to be oriented to the reality of his own body. He has to be reasonably aware of what is happening around him and be sufficiently organized to remain in the dance therapy room.

These patients often have very bizarre, fragmented movements that frequently indicate their own fragmented feelings. One may have to start with a basic exercise such as a patient feeling his feet on the floor. Gradually a patient can feel his whole body to understand that his body is intact and not distorted. During dance therapy an effort is also made to help orient the patient to other people. Sometimes we can deal directly with the bizarre, fragmented movements and ask the patient to interpret his own movements and his own feelings;

□ music therapy is structured reality, derived from tender emotions. When a schizophrenic patient enters a new and perhaps threatening environment we accept him and permit him to trust, share, relate, and organize. The schizophrenic patient has an opportunity to organize around music and to relate to others in a nonverbal manner. It is interesting to note that some schizophrenics cannot speak an organized sentence but can sing an entire song with appropriate feelings.

Sometimes music is the only safe place they can find and the only place they can organize. The music is generally nonthreatening and helps them tune into the world in a group setting. Because music itself has a definite structure, the rhythm alone can help a highly disorganized schizophrenic begin to organize. As the patient progresses we will teach him special musical skills but always in a group situation where two or more patients are taking lessons from the therapist. This enables him to become closer to others without being excessively threatened.

PARTIAL HOSPITALIZATION/OUTPATIENT CARE

When the patient is organized, in control of himself, relating distinctly better to other people, adjusted on medication, and having a reasonably good relationship to his psychotherapist, he is then ready for partial hospitalization or outpatient care. Very frequently the patient must be situated in a halfway house or a living arrangement separate from his disturbed family. Termination should be a warm experience and very often our patients will bake a cake and arrange a farewell party for the patient with all those staff members present who have dealt with the patient during his acute illness.

It is usually best if the patient can continue with the psychiatrist who has treated him in the hospital. We limit our patients to a maximum of two return visits to the psychiatric unit after his hospitalization. These visits are limited to the standard visiting hours.

CONCLUSION

We believe that the utilization of a total, humane, caring therapeutic approach will best enable the patient to function in a happier, more effective manner. Such an approach revolves around the use of family therapy, individual psychotherapy, the necessary pharmacological intervention, group therapy, all of the activities therapies plus the preparation for proper aftercare, followed by individual psychotherapy, proper adjustment of medication, a constructive living environment, and continuing family therapy. In this way the need for another short-term or long-term hospitalization for another acute schizophrenic episode often is precluded.

Theoretical Issues
in Short-Term Treatment

Alan I. Levenson, MD

I am pleased to present the practical aspects of short-term in-patient care as well as its theoretical aspects. All too often, I am afraid, we get so immersed in our day-to-day practical operations that we forget about the theoretical foundations that underlie what we are doing. When this happens, of course, we lose much of the professional satisfaction that comes from understanding what it is that we do and why it is that we do it. At the same time, by forgetting about our theoretical foundations, I am afraid that we severely limit both our own personal productivity and the effectiveness of our methods of practice.

During the past 30 years, short-term inpatient programs have become well established in both general hospital and psychiatric hospital settings. During this time, we have also come a long way in formulating the theoretical basis of this short-term inpatient work. Several basic concepts are essential to our understanding of short-term inpatient care. One of the most basic, in my judgment, relates to the place of short-term inpatient care within the total spectrum of psychiatric services. We know that different patients need different types of care, and we also know that any one patient is likely to need different types of treatment during the course of his illness. For the occasional patient, short-term inpatient care may be the only mode of care that is required for effective and definitive treatment of the

Dr. Levenson is professor and head of the department of psychiatry, University of Arizona, College of Medicine, and is president of the Palo Verde Foundation for Mental Health.

This article was originally published in the National Association of Private Psychiatric Hospitals Journal, Volume 9, Number 1, and is reprinted here with the permission of the publisher.

illness; but for most patients, a period of short-term inpatient care is one part of the total treatment program.

THE CONTINUUM OF PSYCHIATRIC CARE

In a more general sense, short-term inpatient care is one very important part of the total spectrum of comprehensive psychiatric services. Obviously, other parts of this comprehensive spectrum include long-term inpatient, outpatient, and day hospital care. Each of these forms of care has a place in our total treatment programs, and it seems clear that no one of them can stand alone. Each is part of the continuum of psychiatric care; it must always be our goal to make use of each of these elements of care in a manner that is both timely and specific to the needs of our patients.

There are two sides to the emphasis on this continuum. On the one hand, we must keep in mind that short-term inpatient care alone is not the answer to every patient's needs. On the other hand, we must remember that outpatient care is not enough for many patients. While many patients are able to benefit from outpatient care alone, there are many others for whom it is vital that there is a short period of intensive treatment within a hospital setting. Unfortunately, I think, there are some mental health workers and some interested lay people who have tended to overemphasize the significance of outpatient care and to de-emphasize the value of inpatient care. Some have supposedly done this under the banner of community psychiatry, but in doing so, they have forgotten that a basic tenet of community psychiatry is the emphasis on the continuum of services, rather than on emphasis on any one service at the expense of others.

I am afraid that people who emphasize only outpatient care as the basis of community psychiatry have sadly forgotten that short-term inpatient care itself is truly a community psychiatry approach. Unlike the older and more traditional long-term hospitalization programs, short-term hospital care makes it possible for the patient to be treated without being isolated from other members of his family. Short-term inpatient care also lets patients be treated without disruption of ties to work, friends, and the larger community. And, short-term inpatient care makes it possible for the patient to be treated without incurring enormous expense for self, family, or insurance carriers. In these respects, short-term inpatient care has many of the same advantages as community-based outpatient care; but, in addition, short-term inpatient treatment provides for an intensity of care and a variety of treatment modalities that simply cannot be provided outside the hospital environment.

CRISIS THEORY IN SHORT-TERM TREATMENT

I would like to address one of the theoretical concepts that has served a most important basis for the development of specific treatment programs within the hospital setting. Many elements have gone into the development of short-term inpatient treatment programs; but, at least in my judgment, one of the most significant concepts has been that of crisis theory. It has been of great value in many aspects of modern psychiatric practice, and one of these clearly has been the provision of short-term hospital care for acutely ill patients.

The development of crisis theory began with the research of Eric Lindemann (1) at the Massachusetts General Hospital in Boston. Lindemann's work was started in the 1940s and focused on the analysis of emotional reactions to acutely and severely stressful situations, such as his study of survivors of a massive nightclub fire at Boston's Coconut Grove. Lindemann was soon joined in his original studies by Gerald Caplan, and Caplan's writings quickly became preeminent in the crisis theory literature.

Put very simply, a crisis in the sense we are discussing it refers to any emotionally stressful personal experience. Caplan has provided us with a much more detailed definition, and, from my own experience, I think that it is a very useful one for our work in short-term inpatient settings.

He has defined crisis in terms of the problems regularly and naturally faced in the course of daily life. Most of these problems are handled quite satisfactorily and they are readily resolved; but sometimes, of course, they are not. Caplan (2) has described the situation in the following way:

> The essential factor influencing the occurrence of a crisis is an imbalance between the difficulty and importance of the problem (on the one hand) and the resouces immediately available to deal with it. The usual homeostatic, direct problem-solving mechanisms do not work, and the problem is such that other methods that might be used to side step it also cannot be used.

In other words, the problem is one where the individual is faced by stimuli which signal danger to a fundamental need satisfaction or evoke major need appetite, and the circumstances are such that habitual problem-solving methods are unsuccessful within the time span of past expectations of success. Therefore, tension due to frustration of need arises, and this in itself involves problems in maintaining the integrity of the organism or group and may be associated with feelings of subjective discomfort or strain.

THE VALUE OF EARLY INTERVENTION

As Caplan and others have pointed out, a crisis is not necessarily an accidental occurrence; some crises are natural occurrences that are experienced by everyone. These include what Erik Erikson referred to as the "developmental crises," those transitional situations of life that are known to all of us, for example, the death of a loved one or an adolescent's leaving home for college. Clearly, these situations are common, if not universal; but individual reactions to these situations vary tremendously. Most people handle such crises quite successfully. In terms of Caplan's model, they find adequate resources in family, friends, and community to help solve the problem even though they have never faced anything like it before. For psychiatrists and others in the mental health field, the focus of clinical concern is the other group—those who have not only been unable to cope with the crisis but also have developed a mental illness as a result. Atlthough it may well be obvious to all of us, I think it most important that we always remember that a mental illness may be seen in the context of either type of crisis—the unexpected accidental one or the natural developmental one. Both are potentially very dangerous, and either can lead to a severe mental disorder.

Crisis theory offers much to help us in understanding the nature of an acute mental illness and the circumstances of its onset. Crisis theory also helps us in the development of effective treatment programs for these acute illnesses.

One of the principal lessons of crisis theory is that early treatment is usually the most effective. Early intervention is the key, then, to effective treatment; but, to be effective, treatment efforts must be specific and intensive. In many instances only a short-term inpatient setting can provide the necessary level of care for an acutely mentally ill patient.

Short-term therapy is a crisis intervention approach; as such, it is not intended to be used as a means of transforming or rebuilding a patient's total personality. Rather, short-term inpatient care, like all crisis-intervention methods, is oriented toward restoring the patient to his premorbid level of functioning. This type of treatment provides an effective means of helping the patient to prepare for dealing successfuly with new crises in the future, but it leaves the restructuring of basic personality factors for subsequent care—usually provided on an outpatient basis over a long period of time, if it is to be provided at all.

MILIEU THERAPY

In the minds of some people, this type of specific goal-oriented inpatient treatment may seem too limited, but, in reality, the goal directedness of the therapy is one of its great strengths. Patients are provided with quick and effective relief; expensive hospital resources are used only to provide services for which they are specifically needed. Many patients may well need treatment beyond that for the immediate crisis, but this can typically be provided with equal effectiveness and with much lower cost on an outpatient basis. As a result, the period of inpatient care can be limited to treatment that, on the one hand, is oriented toward resolving the acute problem and, on the other hand, is oriented toward providing the patient with a period of transition to longer term outpatient care.

The concepts of crisis theory are some of the most helpful in our theoretical understanding of short-term inpatient care. Another concept that has great significance is that of milieu therapy, or, as many people prefer to describe it, the therapeutic community. It really does not matter which term is used; what counts is the principle and the approach of carefully structuring every aspect of inpatient program functions so that each one makes a positive contribution to the treatment process.

The concept of milieu therapy carries with it the proposition that everything that happens in the inpatient setting has an effect on the patient and on his therapeutic progress. The milieu therapy approach, however, goes much beyond this simple expectation of effect: the real essence of milieu therapy is the idea that the inpatient environment can be intentionally controlled and consciously manipulated to have a planned and specified effect on each patient. In many nonpsychiatric settings, the hospital environment is simply a diffuse background for the implementation of specific diagnostic and treatment procedures. But, in the setting of the short-term psychiatric inpatient program, the hospital environment itself becomes a critical element in that diagnostic and treatment process.

The concept of milieu therapy is based in large part on the premise that an inpatient psychiatric unit is a social system. As such, its operation is directly influenced by the patients and the staff who are the members of this social system, and it is influenced further by the physical and organizational surroundings of the inpatient unit.

In theoretical terms, the operation and effectiveness of milieu therapy can be easily described and readily understood. Robert Daniels (3) has pointed out that we can use both psychodynamic and behavioral formulations to explain the process of milieu therapy or therapeutic community. He writes:

> In the psychodynamic, psychoanalytic framework, hypotheses about the therapeutic effects of the therapeutic community center on the interface between ego functions and environment. The environment may alter or shape certain psychodynamic balances that are intrapsychic. Some of these structures or functions are the adaptive functions of the ego, ego defenses, the self-systems, and object representations. The inputs from the environment of the hospital ward are intended to provide predictability, certainty, and continuity of experience for the patient, thereby reducing anxiety, guilt, and shame. The corrective experience of an environment that is more reality oriented and is humane, promotes the reduction of these painful tensions and the associated structural and economic imbalances. If successful, the therapeutic community promotes more appropriate and more realistic interpersonal relations. It enhances self-esteem and reduces feelings of wrongdoing or sinfulness. These changes in intrapsychic factors, chiefly in the ego, allow the patient's healthier adaptive capacities to reassert themselves. Often, there is a snowball effect in which multiple inputs affecting various systems—biological systems, social systems, and psychological systems—combine to promote a better adaptive state.
>
> The therapeutic community offers opportunities to influence and shape behavior through systems of rewards and punishment, both overt and covert. To the extent that such interven-

tions are consciously undertaken—that is, planned, executed, and evaluated—they may be thought of as theoretical and therapeutic extensions of behavioral therapy. Whether consciously intended or not, however, they exist; one cannot structure a social system without having many such influences. Therapeutic decisions about privileges, constraints, and discharge may be viewed by the staff and the patients as rewards or punishments. As such, they may influence behavior in desired therapeutic outcomes, or they may become antitherapeutic if applied in an arbitrary or authoritarian fashion. Thus, almost every therapeutic community uses some therapeutic elements of psychoanalytic understanding and some elements of behavioral understanding.

The development of a therapeutic milieu is a tremendously important part of a short-term inpatient program. Without it, an inpatient unit is likely to produce what is actually an antitherapeutic effect. The typical hospital environment is one that promotes dependence and regression on the part of the patient; and, in the absence of careful attention to the therapeutic milieu, the typical patient is placed in an infantilized role. The first goal of a therapeutic milieu, then, is to prevent regressive behavior that intensifies the patient's illness; and, as a substitute for unnatural and overdrawn dependency, the therapeutic milieu encourages of even forces the patient to become an active, independent participant in his own treatment.

Any hospital admission will necessarily bring about some degree of passivity and regression on the part of the patient. To some extent this is what has been called "regression in the service of the ego"; as such, it is a necessary and positive component of the treatment process. At the same time, however, regression that is uncontrolled and outside the context of the total treatment program becomes destructive rather than constructive; the therapeutic milieu is designed to make a regression—like all other aspects of the patient's behavior—a positive rather than a negative experience.

Milieu therapy also has the tremendous value of providing a setting in which a very wide range of treatment modalities can be brought to bear. Both psychodynamically oriented and behaviorally oriented treatment approaches become increasingly effective in milieu therapy. Individual psychotherapy, group therapy, family therapy, desensitization procedures, implosive therapy—all have a place within the context of a short-term inpatient unit. In addition the use of a wide variety of medications and other somatic methods, like electroconvulsive therapy, is equally important in the treatment of patients in a short-term inpatient unit; their effectiveness and value are enhanced when prescribed in a milieu therapy program.

Although many aspects of a short-term inpatient psychiatric program are worthy of discussion, I have touched on only a few of them in terms of the theoretical aspects of such a program. There are two other closely related concepts that are particularly significant in short-term inpatient work and, as such, need to be at least briefly mentioned. The first of these is the vital importance of having a multidisciplinary staff team for the development and operation of a short-term inpatient unit; the second corollary issue is the importance of providing medical direction for this team.

As I have tried to indicate, a successful short-term inpatient program must be able to provide a wide variety of services and must be able to meet a wide variety of patient needs. It should not seem too surprising, then, that the successful short-term inpatient program must be staffed by people who bring many different perspectives to bear on the treatment being provided for each patient. Psychiatry, psychology, social work, and psychiatric nursing are typically thought of as the four core mental health professional disciplines. All four must be represented on the staff of the short-term inpatient unit; and, in addition, vital contributions can be made by professionals in such fields as occupational, activity, music, dance, and art therapies. In addition, an essential place on the multidisciplinary hospital staff team is available for many paraprofessionals and nonprofessionals.

The essential treatment medium in a short-term psychiatric inpatient unit is, quite simply, people. In terms that economists like to use, the human orientation of our work makes our field probably the most "labor intensive" of all branches of medicine; and, the many people who provide the services of a short-term psychiatric inpatient unit can be effective only when they are drawn from many different fields and are functioning as members of an integrated team.

A SPECIAL ROLE

This general idea is probably obvious to all who have any knowledge of short-term inpatient units and their methods of successful operation. What often seems less obvious, however, is the fact that the multidisciplinary team approach does not mean that everyone on the team performs the same function. The team concept implies that many people are working together in a coordinated fashion and with a common goal; but it also implies that each member of the team has a set of specific, differentiated tasks that he must perform. The existence of a team approach does not mean that everyone does the same thing; and, although there will be some overlapping functions within the team, the approach does not mean blurring of the team members' roles. Every member of the team must have specific functions to perform; otherwise, the team will not succeed in its common task.

A discussion of staff roles within the inpatient unit team immediately brings up the question of the special role—and the special responsibilities—of the physician member of that team. Any discussion of the physician's role introduces the matter that is generally referred to as the issue of the "medical model." The present concept of short-term inpatient care includes the expectation—and indeed the requirement—that a physician will assume responsibility for the overall direction and coordination of the psychiatric services within a hospital. Although this approach is well established, there are many who have long questioned the preeminence of the medical model in our approach to the care of the mentally ill and, in so doing, have questioned the role of the psychiatrist as the physician responsible for the patient's care.

Every theory must be constantly open to question and examination. This scrutiny must be undertaken both by those who endorse the theory and those who deny its validity. It is my own personal view that when questions were first asked about the medical model and its validity, these questions were raised in a spirit of substantive inquiry and examination. But it is also my view that, like so many other things in today's world, the concern for this substantive review and consideration has been overshadowed by issues of interprofessional politics and interdisciplinary rivalries. I find it hard to view the matter in any other way when the issue is removed from the realm of discussion among mental health professionals and transferred to the judicial processes of the courtroom and the quasijudicial proceedings of federal regulatory agencies.

The essence of the medical model, of course, is the simple premise that mental disorders are to be treated as illnesses. Although those who argue against this premise suggest that this kind of categorization is too narrow, I think that the classification of these disorders as illnesses provides a broad and unrestricted approach to their treatment. Illness is generally defined as an absence of health or a deviation from the normal state that we consider to be healthy. The World Health Organization defines health as "a state of complete, mental and social well being . . . ." If anything is wrong with that definition of health, and by extrapolation its corollary definition of illness, surely it must be that the definition is too broad and not that it is too narrow. Our approach to the understanding and treatment of a mental disorder is certainly much enhanced by this broadly based definition.

About ten years ago Ralph M. Kaufman (4) then the Chairman of the Department of Psychiatry at Mount Sinai Hospital in New York, published a paper in which he suggested that there is no one medical model but, rather, multiple medical models. His thesis is generally accepted in medicine: the physician must be concerned with the biological, psychological, and social aspects of the patient's disorder; and, moreover, factors in any or all of these three areas are likely to play a part in the etiology, course, treatment, and outcome of the patient's illness.

CONCLUSION

The physician brings the broad outlook to the care of the patient; and for this reason the medical model—or medical models as Kaufman would put it—places the overall control of that care in the physician's hands. According to this same medical model, the physician also brings a unique sense of responsibility to the care of the patient. Many who object to the primacy of the physician and the dominance of the medical model have argued that the patient himself is responsible for getting better and that the therapist's only role is to serve as a catalyst or helper in this self-treatment process. In other words, they argue that the medical model does not apply in cases of mental illness because it is up to the patient—not the therapist—to "do something" to resolve the patient's problem. This approach, of course, clearly overlooks the fact that responsibility for "doing something" is shared by both physician and patient in most illnesses. It is true, of course, that the surgeon "does something" both for and to the patient with acute appendicitis; but it is also true that the patient has as much responsibility as does the physician in assuring effective treatment in cases of cardiac disease, hypertension, and diabetes—to name a few examples.

Once upon a time, it may have been easy to separate theoretical and practical issues. Certainly, the consideration of theoretical concerns has some value as an intellectual exercise; but, our principal concern must be the care of patients and, as a result, our principal focus must be on the practice of clinical psychiatry. As a result, excursions into the realm of theory should have some practical utility.

REFERENCES

1. Lindemann, E. I. 1944. Symptomatology and management of acute grief. *The Amer. J. of Psychiat.* 101: 141-48.

2. Caplan, G. 1964. *Principles of preventive psychiatry.* New York: Basic Books.

3. Daniels, R. S. 1975. The hospital as a therapeutic community. *The Comprehensive textbook of psychiatry.* 2nd ed. eds. A. M. Freedman, H. I. Kaplan, and B. J. Sadock, pp. 1990-95. Baltimore: Williams and Wilkins.

4. Kaufman, R. M. 1967. Psychiatry—Why 'medical' or 'social' model. *Arch. Gen. Psychiat.* 17: 347-60.

A Psychiatrist's Experience
with Occupational Therapy
in a Short-Term General Hospital Unit

Marc Hertzman, MD

ABSTRACT. Occupational therapy and psychiatry are natural allies. They come at the patient from different points of view, but with similar aims. Each must learn enough of the other's discipline to ask the right questions.

Mutual staff support promotes effective patient care. In psychiatry co-therapy can provide such support. It is possible to enhance reciprocal respect through clear, frank, frequent feedback. Where collegial relationships are inherently unequal, special attention must be paid to finding appropriate forms and ways to anticipate and resolve conflict.

Interdisciplinary collaboration in its finest sense means that professionals with varying types of degrees and training work together for the common good. Mental health has a long and distinguished history of contributions to models of interdisciplinary collaboration. Indeed, it may be fair to say that mental health has led other health fields into this arena. In part the press for defining areas of special expertise or function has been a practical one. Psychiatric patients have long outnumbered other types of patients in the health care inpatient systems, and this remains true even though the focus of hospitalization has shifted to general hospital care. There has been more than enough work to go around, and too few to do it. Notwithstanding a heavy investment of Federal and other dollars in mental health care, the relative dearth of willing professionals, as compared to other service fields, remains.

Dr. Hertzman is Associate Professor and Director of Inpatient Services, Department of Psychiatry and Behavioral Sciences, George Washington University Medical Center, 2150 Pennsylvania Avenue, N.W., Washington, D.C. 20037.

101

Occupational therapy and psychiatry, in particular, have much to offer each other. The main foci of the two professions are distinctly different, although overlapping. That is, occupational therapy tends to stress everyday function, whereas psychiatry most frequently concerns itself with the understanding and modification of patients' inner lives and external modes of communication. In fact, psychiatry is ultimately aimed at function, too, but, in practice, works on helping patients arrive there by somewhat different means. In other words, the outcome goals of the two professions coincide to a relatively high degree, but the therapeutic work may be stressing different routes to arrive there.

TOWARDS CLOSER WORKING RELATIONSHIPS

Occupational therapy and psychiatry are natural allies. Hard times in health and social program funding are presently making it more important for mental health disciplines to work together, instead of engaging in the divisive kind of back biting that fuels outside critics in their efforts to cut back treatment for psychiatric patients. In this respect, occupational therapy as a discipline has taken quite constructive measures. For one, the utility of a profession has to be articulated, demonstrated as scientifically as possible, and set forth for the consuming public to understand. A framework for doing just that appears to be evolving in occupational therapy, using systems concepts, and has been elaborated (Kielhofner, 1980). The language is familiar to social scientists of many stripes, including social psychiatrists.

For present purposes, a straightforward scheme of an inpatient psychiatric system may assist in our orientation (Figure 1). The system is patient-centered, rather than staff, group, or family centered. However the ward staff will be strongly influenced by the extent to which a hospitalization is therapeutic for patients and their families. The staff will be much better equipped to resolve patients' conflicts if they have done significant work upon their own staff subsystem problems.

> A 17-year-old brittle diabetic was admitted to the hospital with frequent episodes of overdosing herself on insulin. Her parents were in despair, and at loggerheads with each other as to what to do. A similar scenario was reenacted in the hospital when the patient's nurse and an occupational therapist disagreed

about her activity schedule. Each complained to the unit director-psychiatrist, rather than to each other. The director initially took sides, but later sat the various staff members down together to agree on an approach to the patient. In the course of the discussion, it gradually became clear that each discipline felt it should have priority access to the patient. The staff as a group, thus alerted, later went on to set some general priorities for scheduling patient's activities.

While there is some risk of occupational therapy identifying too closely with a wing of psychiatry that is in eclipse at this time, i.e. social and community psychiatry, if the product being propounded is basically sound, it should ultimately emerge for what it is worth.

Figure 1. Patient-Centered Ward Subsystems*

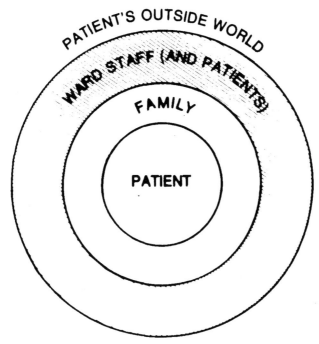

*Modified from Hertzman, M. *Restoring Function Rapidly.* New York, Human Sciences Press, forthcoming.

Conversely, assertions based upon faith alone will likely convince few, friends or skeptics, that occupation therapy is essential and important to patient care. In the main, occupational therapy appears to be on the right track towards putting itself on a firm utilitarian basis. In order to be firmly ensconced in general hospitals, occupational therapy must prove that it is essential. An example is that of determining which items of information need to be documented systematically, and in what ways, in order to deliver high quality care, increase the likelihood of reimbursability, and pass accreditation inspections. Occupational therapy has been instrumental, for instance, in getting the Joint Commission on Accreditation of Hospitals to include elements of occupational therapy as requirements needing to be met for hospitals' accreditation awards.

Psychiatry has come increasingly to recognize its debt to occupational therapy, also. The last edition of the diagnostic Bible, the *Diagnostic and Statistical Manual-III* of the American Psychiatric Association, incorporates two different classification schemata (American Psychiatric Association, 1980). The text, too, takes a longitudinal view of how patients function in their everyday lives, in determining the likelihood of various diagnoses like schizophrenia. This convergence between occupational therapy and psychiatric conceptualizations is surely more than accidental.

Stating the case for interdisciplinary collaboration inevitably leads to some distortions, usually of the idealized kind. When collaboration is working well, it is fulfilling; when the participants are not collaborating, it can be worse than working alone. To understand just how well occupational therapists and psychiatrists can work together in practice requires another level of analysis. It requires some dissection of professional role functions, and of responsibility relationships. These are discussed hereafter as a succession of triangulations among communications. First is the direct work with the patient. Next is support among staff, most particularly on a psychiatric inpatient unit. Then, there are the interactions among each other, occupational therapists, psychiatrists, and other staff.

CARRYING OUT THERAPY

Therapy is taking place when efforts are evolving to change someone's state for the presumptive better. Occupational therapy and psychiatry both presume at least an initial push from someone other than the patient, and usually one that continues for some time. In order for this to proceed, an elaboration of the problems must occur, the evaluation, which is hopefully therapeutic in and of itself. For the present discussion, it is assumed that the basic elements of a psychiatric and occupational therapy assessment are well-known. It is our observation that occupational therapy personnel generally have a much better idea of the psychiatric evaluation than vice-versa. This is one of a number of examples of crucial junctures where communication is weighted in a one-sided manner. Since power and authority generally rest with the psychiatrist for both the patient's care, and programs as well, the typical occupational therapist is situated in a delicate position. To presume too much is likely to result in being dismissed as pushy and over-aggressive. On the other hand, timidity or overrestraint in proactive communication towards the psychiatrist is likewise an invitation to feeling shunted aside and unappreciated for one's contributions. Furthermore, it is frustrating and tiring to find oneself saying the same things repeatedly about different, or even the same patients.

Small wonder, then, that, in our program, occupational therapists have developed into the prime promoters of assertiveness training. This type of therapy was introduced as a high-level group series of exercises for patients close to leaving the hospital. In this guise, not only has it been not-threatening, but other professional staff have been quick to realize its potential for improving their own affectually laden communication skills, and have requested of occupational therapy that staff training and workshops be available in assertiveness training.

This is one example of a constructive spinoff from an accurate analysis of difficulties in interdisciplinary role function. As a general strategy it suggests that demonstration of effectiveness is worth a thousand words of explanation. Moreover, it seems likely that disciplines working together need constantly to reorient themselves to their roles as gentle teachers of one another. Here the role may not be explicitly conferred, but takes place *de facto*. Once it starts to work well, the inexplicit nature of it can, much more acceptably, be regularized in an open, mutually beneficial way.

More than anything else, direct patient care demands being able to form a relationship with the patient. In general hospital care, where there is a premium upon finishing the bulk of the work within days to weeks, there may not be much leisure to allow professional/patient relationships to develop gradually. Thus the choice upon whom among the professional staff the patient bestows his trust may not precisely fit the prescribed order in the treatment plan. It then becomes a matter of the staff's adapting to the patient and working through that professional staff member who holds the patient's trust more closely.

> W.E. was a brilliant schizophrenic in his late forties, whose illness had severely limited his functional adjustment throughout his life. He was chronically incapacitated, spending long periods in the hospital, and living a marginal existence in the community for varying lengths of time in between these. When admitted to the hospital, he was quite delusional, in a bizarre, outspoken, and sometimes aggressive way. His psychiatrist, a private practitioner, and he were currently having trouble agreeing on anything.
>
> Among the other modalities of treatment, W.E. was referred to individual occupational therapy assessment, and whatever else might help. The occupational therapist diagnosed difficulties in going from abstract to concrete, and outlined a regimen of individual projects to be undertaken on a regular schedule with her direct assistance. The patient was enthusiastic, participatory, and easily engageable. It became quickly clear to the occupational therapist that their budding relationship had much to do with the patient's sexual attraction to her, and probably little to do with his intrinsic motivation for the tasks. Nevertheless, hers was one of the few positive relationships W.E. was having at the time, and that recognition made it possible to build upon their work and extend it to include psychiatry.

It is also clear that there is great potential for conflict here. The two professional were in positions vis-à-vis the patient where it is easy for jealously, competition, and rivalry, stimulated unwittingly by the patient, to supercede collaboration. Moreover, some schizophrenics, like borderline patients are capable of "splitting," unconsciously, through their behavior; exploiting and exposing latent staff conflicts. This type of situation is a real test of the maturity and selflessness of the professionals involved.

SUPPORTING STAFF

The previous examples should already make it clear how important it can be for disciplines to support each other. But what does "support" mean? Some elements are more useful to the maintenance of morale and furthering of psychiatric work than others. They include listening empathically, being able to challenge another's distortions in ways that will ultimately be possible for the other to incorporate. Confirmation of one's beliefs in the notion that one has done an effective job with the patient is probably the most important support that can be rendered, one staff member to another. This includes being explicit about what actions should be repeated, done more vigorously, differently, or not at all. Support needs to be initiated and carried out repeatedly and exhaustively, because it is so difficult to sustain working with psychiatric inpatients for any length of time. Nonetheless, it is non-supportive to do it with false praise. This only entrenches the recipient staff member in unproductive routines.

Support needs to be seen as reciprocal. This can be particularly likely to be practiced in the breach because of the unbalanced positions of authority on an inpatient service, such as those between occupational therapy and psychiatry. They are not insurmountable, however, over the long haul, with professionals, motivated to try. On both sides the issues boil down to learning to recognize the job well done as it is happening, and exercising the ability to articulate this as close to the events as possible. Indeed, since this may be the heart of what patients need to learn to do in therapy for themselves, it is reasonable for the staff to demand no less from themselves.

In our program occupational therapy has been particularly influential in suggesting how group therapies should be run. The organizational structure of the group has been described elsewhere in systems terms (Hertzman, Hertzman, and Kaplan). The groups are arranged hierarchically by level of functions (Figure 2). They can also be conceputalized as ministering to patient needs on a series of continua (Figure 3). Thus, patients have an individual treatment plan tailored for them that takes into account both their global abilities to adapt, and specific problem areas upon which they may be focusing. One effective way of structuring the work so as to promote such support is to set out deliberately to conduct much of the therapeutic work with co-therapists for different disciplines.

A by-product of the systems design on the unit is a group targeted for quite low-functioning patient's defined operationally as those who can, at a minimum, remain in the same (closed) room with half a dozen patients for a minimum of five to ten minutes (Kaplan, 1980). These are patients who are usually psychotic, or recently so, severely depressed to the point of inanition, or significantly im-

FIGURE 2.*

FRAMEWORK OF THE GROUP TREATMENT PROGRAM

I. HIERARCHICAL STRUCTURE

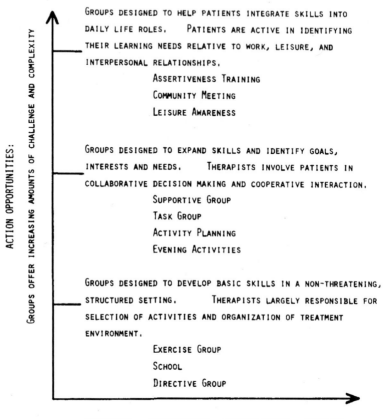

COGNITIVE   INTERPERSONAL   PSYCHOLOGICAL   PHYSICAL

INDIVIDUAL SKILLS AND PERFORMANCE CAPABILITIES

*From Hertzman, Hertzman, and Kaplan, 1983

paired cognitively. This group is co-lead by an occupational therapist and a psychiatrist.

Co-leadership allows the professionals to solidify their understanding of how the groups are working, and intensifies staff
awareness of the need for inservice training and supervision on technique. The main staff work on being mutually supportive is carried

FIGURE 3. *

II. HORIZONTAL DIMENSION: WIDE RANGE OF NEEDS ADDRESSED

DAILY OCCUPATION

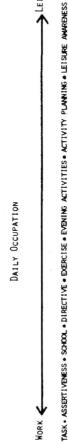

WORK ⟷ LEISURE

TASK • ASSERTIVENESS • SCHOOL • DIRECTIVE • EXERCISE • EVENING ACTIVITIES • ACTIVITY PLANNING • LEISURE AWARENESS

EMOTIONAL/PHYSICAL WELL-BEING

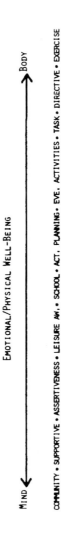

MIND ⟷ BODY

COMMUNITY • SUPPORTIVE • ASSERTIVENESS • LEISURE AW. • SCHOOL • ACT. PLANNING • EVE. ACTIVITIES • TASK • DIRECTIVE • EXERCISE

INTERPERSONAL RELATIONSHIPS

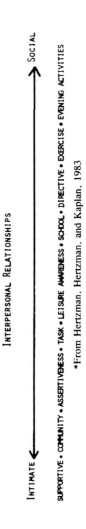

INTIMATE ⟷ SOCIAL

SUPPORTIVE • COMMUNITY • ASSERTIVENESS • TASK • LEISURE AWARENESS • SCHOOL • DIRECTIVE • EXERCISE • EVENING ACTIVITIES

*From Hertzman, Hertzman, and Kaplan, 1983

out in planning and posting the group each day. It may even take several years of working together before each co-leader knows what to expect from the other. Longstanding relationships facilitate constructive criticism, to be sure, but it is equally clear that only frankness with each other has allowed the professional to develop the group—and themselves—over time. For example, the first year of running the group for low-functioning patients was basically one of trials and errors, until a format was achieved which took cognizance of the functional capabilities of the patients on a variety of continua: cognitive, gross and fine motor, social skills, initiative abilities, and the like. It will immediately be apparent to occupational therapists that this is the language to which they are accustomed. Curiously, however, in the developmental history of the group, it may have been the psychiatrist who first emphasized the need for an active, directing, structured staff input to the patients. The mutuality has resulted in a pleasant, often teasing atmosphere, in which both therapists strongly accentuate for the patients what they can do, and de-emphasize litanies of despair.

Much staff support comes in the form of didactic education. A particularly effective contribution that occupational therapy can make is to set up and carry out active training exercises for the staff which require integrating thought, feeling, and action. Psychiatry and occupational therapy together can assure that all staff orientations include these elements. This is especially germane each time there is staff turnover, or, as is the case on a training unit, when new students arrive. We have found that catching new staff, of all disciplines, at the earliest possible moment in their arrival on the unit is most likely to optimize teaching impact, as measured by their subsequent behaviors. The occupational therapy staff will usually ask them to participate in exercises that they will later be able to use with patients, acclimatizing them not only by lecturing, but by hands-on sensory experiences of therapeutic-like sessions.

RESOLVING INTERDISCIPLINARY CONFLICTS

We have already alluded to some of the myriads of possible interdisciplinary interactions that bear directly upon inpatient mental health work. In the event that it is not clear, we shall restate the following: the object of interdisciplinary collaboration should always be to turn potential conflict into complementarity. "Con-

flict'' is disagreement, in action. By ''complementarity'' we mean
''constructive resolution of conflict that enhances goal-directed
work, and eventually contributes to mutual respect.'' Note that conflicts may not be resolvable at times without some residual feelings
of anger, defeat, and so on. Smoothing ruffled feathers, however,
does not necessarily lead to optimizing decisions.

> For more than a year staff members had been undercutting
> each other on carrying out agreed-upon patient treatment
> plans. A typical response when a staff member would be con-
> fronted with such behavior was to respond, ''I didn't under-
> stand the treatment plan.'' It required many staff meetings for
> the director to realize that this translated into the tacit cor-
> ollary, ''If I don't understand it, I don't have to do it.'' From
> this point on, staff members of various disciplines were re-
> quired to summarize their understanding of treatment plans,
> out loud and on paper before they left each team meeting.

The management of conflict resolution has been studied exten-
sively, especially by specialists in organizational development.
Veniga has provided a useful elaboration of approaches to dealing
with conflict (Veniga, 1979). Like Filley (1975), Veniga suggests
that consensus strategies which may be lowest common de-
nominator solutions, are sub-optimal. He has provided a systematic
approach to the processes, which is summarized in Table 1. Certain
skills that occupational therapy practitioners acquire in their training—as do a number of other disciplines—are particularly germane.
These include articulating a clear definition of roles on the ward and
using adult interpersonal relations in the service of problem solving.
It is not difficult to recognize conflict when it erupts. The art of
working together is to anticipate it at early stages, long before the
volcano has had a chance to begin to smolder. An essential element
for identifying conflict early on, or the potential for it, is to provide
and take advantage of many opportunities for face-to-face exchange.
This works best by far when it is done in pairs, and privately. The
heyday of therapeutic communities has left a certain mark on many
inpatient services. The notion often exists that all things can be
shared openly by all people, in all forums. (This is exaggeration to
make a point.) In fact, it is much easier to accept criticism, especially negative, but even positive, when it is done tactfully, and
with a minimum of shaming. A particularly unconstructive place for

TABLE 1.*

AN APPROACH TO CONFLICT RESOLUTION

. Recognize that a serious problem of disagreement exists.

. Determine the optimal groups of person, time, and place to begin resolution.

. Define the problem. Include feelings and attitudes.

. Identify alternative solutions.

. Weight advantages and limitations of each.

. Determine support for the plan.

. Implement the plan. Decide how the outcome will be evaluated.

. Evaluate the plan.

*Modified from Veniga, 1979

confrontation, for example, is a staff meeting. However useful such meetings may be for identifying who is in conflict with whom, and over what, they are not the places to settle things.

The implication of this stance is that frequent, regular collaborative and supervisory meetings need to be scheduled. The psychiatrist has a supervisory responsibility towards occupational therapy in most psychiatric hospital ward settings. This needs to be exercised actively, not left to happenstance, which only leads to "management by exception," recognition of the supervisee's work only at time of failure. The latter is a surefire formula for staff demoralization.

How is it possible to expect mutuality, respect, feedback, and support, if the relationships are inherently unequal? This is a dilemma that surely applies to many experiences that each person has throughout life in many settings. There are no easy answers, but there are some ways of working on the problem, continually, that seem to contribute more than others.

One concrete example is a set of written expectations for job performance, as specific as possible. Once again, this idea tends to be much more than a general job description. The job performance sheet is essentially an outline of what the professional staff members will achieve in the next six months or a year. It includes descriptions of outcome measures, how these are to be achieved, and who will assess the goodness of fit between ideals and actualities along the way. Although it tends to be the supervisor who does the assessing, a clear job performance sheet ought to be readily decipherable to anyone in the field. The process of construction is probably even more important than the content. It begins with the professional's self-assessment, and continues with periodic, frequent feedback about how things are going.

Psychiatrists certainly need feedback, too, about their own performance. When a psychiatrist is the unit director, it is easy for him to become isolated from other staff. The tendency on the part of the staff is to hang back from expressions of positive feedback. Perhaps this is a product of our school training, in which such strokes were considered "applepolish" for the teacher, subject to scorn by one's peers on the playground afterwards. Whatever the sources, and whatever the concerns about glossing over failures and weaknesses on the part of the director, this is a matter that requires constant attention from all disciplines to overcome, because it is basically unhealthy for such a unit.

A related problem is that of two-person discussions about a third party in the latter's absence. The prototype for this is railing about one's relationship with the third party, without dealing directly and coming to some new settlement. Professionals can do each other a great service by insisting upon participating in negatively critical conversations only in the presence of the principals to the acrimony. Nothing is easier to assess as important; nothing harder to do, in practice. Doing so, and insisting on it, far from discouraging open exchange, tends to promote a higher level, growth-promoting discourse on the ward.

REFERENCES

American Psychiatric Association. *Diagnostic and Statistical Manual-III.* Washington, D.C.: APA, 1980.
Filley, A.C. *Interpersonal Conflict Resolution.* Glenview, Ill: Scott Foresman and Co., 1975.
Hertzman, M. *Restoring Function Rapidly.* New York: Human Sciences Press, forthcoming, 1984.

Hertzman, M., Hertzman, R.C., and Kaplan, K. Inpatient group therapy in a short-term general hospital. Presentation at the World Congress of Psychiatry, Vienna, Austria, 1983.

Kaplan, K. Directive Group: Treatment for psychiatric patients with extreme occupational dysfunction. Unpublished Manuscript, 1980.

Keilhofner, G. and Burke, J. A model of human occupation: Part one; conceptual framework, and content. *American Journal of Occupational Therapy.* 34,572-581, 1980.

Veniga, R. The management of disruptive conflicts. *Hospital and Health Services* Administration, 8-29, Spring, 1979.